Multiple Sclerosis

PROGRESS IN REHABILITATION

Multiple Sclerosis

Edited by

Rudy Capildeo
and
Audrey Maxwell

M

First published 1982 by
THE MACMILLAN PRESS LTD.
London and Basingstoke
Companies and representatives throughout the world

Typeset in Baskerville by Multiplex Techniques Ltd,
Orpington, Kent

Printed in Hong Kong

ISBN 0 333 30965 0 (hard cover)
0 333 30966 9 (paper cover)

Contents

The Contributors

R. BEARD, FRCS,
Senior Registrar in Urology, St Thomas' Hospital, London SE1

R. CAPILDEO, MB, BS, MRCP,
Senior Registrar, Department of Neurology, Charing Cross Hospital, London W6

M.A. CRAWFORD, PhD,
Head of Biochemistry Department, Nuffield Laboratories of Comparative Medicine at the Institute of Zoology, London, and Special Professor at the Department of Applied Biochemistry and Nutrition, University of Nottingham

C.D. EVANS, MB, BS, MRCP, DPhys Med, FBIM,
General Practitioner, Purley, Surrey

C. H. HAWKES, BSc, MD, MRCP,
Consultant Neurologist, Ipswich Hospital, Suffolk, and Honorary Clinical Assistant, Institute of Neurology, London

Judith HARDING, BSc (Hons) Nutr, SRD,
ARMS Research Unit, Central Middlesex Hospital, London NW10 7NS

Audrey MAXWELL,
Consultant to *Therapy*, Macmillan Journals, 4 Little Essex St, London WC2R 3LF

Alison PERRY, LCST,
Chief Speech Therapist, Speech Therapy Department, Charing Cross Hospital, London W6

Christine RANDALL,
Training Officer, Surrey Social Services

J. SIMKINS,
Chairman, Action for Research into Multiple Sclerosis, 71 Grays Inn Road, London WC1X 8TR

June SUTHERLAND, Dip COT,
Head Occupational Therapist, Westminster Hospital, London SW1

D.G. THOMAS, MRCP, FRCS,
Senior Lecturer in Neurosurgery and Consultant Neurosurgeon, Institute of Neurology, London WC1

Jennifer TODD, MCSP,
Formerly Superintendent Physiotherapist, Royal Hospital and Home for Incurables, London SW15

Introduction

Rudy Capildeo and Audrey Maxwell

Multiple sclerosis is the commonest neurological disease in Great Britain. But what is multiple sclerosis? The simple answer is that although a great deal is known about the disease, the aetiology remains unknown. An enormous amount of research has been undertaken in the last 20 years and is continuing unabated now, but the benefit for the individual sufferer is hard to demonstrate. However, such has been the progress made in multiple sclerosis research units that many workers in this difficult field believe that a major break-through is imminent.

Until this happens we must continue to look after our patients in the best way that we can, by improving our knowledge of the disease, and by helping patients and relatives to understand it, how we can help them, and how they can help themselves. Still there are too many misconceptions about the disease which must be dispelled.

Rehabilitation begins with the diagnosis of multiple sclerosis. Individual responses, physically and psychologically, vary greatly from patient to patient. In a disease which is so variable, generalisations should be avoided.

The rehabilitation team observes and treats the individual. This approach, that of a multidisciplinary team looking after a patient, means that each member of the team has to be aware of what other members of the team have to offer and can try to achieve. Even those therapists who have no opportunity to work within the framework of a rehabilitation team should know what other disciplines have to offer. They can therefore endeavour to bring together those members of the hospital and community health care teams in order to assess and treat the multiple sclerosis patient as effectively as possible.

Very few medical books have been written for therapists. It is hoped that this book will fill one significant gap. It has been written using the concept of a rehabilitation team. Although the emphasis of the presentation is towards paramedical members of the team, it is hoped that this book will be of use to medical staff, doctors and nurses.

This integrated approach to patient care, we believe, is the basic philosophy of rehabilitation.

1 Medical aspects of multiple sclerosis

Rudy Capildeo

Historical aspects

Multiple sclerosis was first clinically defined by Jean-Martin Charcot in 1868 (Capildeo, 1982). This famous French physician (1825-93) worked at the Salpêtrière, an asylum for over 5000 inmates in Paris. He was to establish the first Chair of Neurology in the world. In addition to his own students, who were to become famous (for example Pierre Marie, Jules Dejerine, Joseph Babinski, Gilles de la Tourette, to name but a few), physicians from other countries came to study under Charcot. In time they would develop neurology as a new speciality in their own countries. Sigmund Freud was amongst these students.

Charcot was the master of clinico-pathological demonstrations - linking the clinical features of a disease with the pathological findings. In his teaching he also enjoyed comparing and contrasting patients with the same disease as well as with different diseases. The novelty of his teaching methods would assure his reputation, but his original contributions, not only in the field of neurology but also within the wider aspects of general medicine (for example gout, tuberculosis, and liver and kidney diseases), and his publications would ensure that Charcot would be remembered as the first and greatest neurologist.

The plaques in the nervous system had been demonstrated by Jean Cruveilhier (1791-1873) and by Robert Carswell (1793-1857), the former a French pathologist, the latter an Aberdeen graduate who became Professor of Pathology at University College, London (1828). Cruveilhier's water-colour studies of diseased structures are famous. Charcot separated multiple sclerosis as a distinct clinical entity from other cases of neurological disease.

It may seem surprising now, but before Charcot the type of tremor seen in multiple sclerosis (intention tremor, absent at rest, appearing during voluntary action) had not been distinguished from the type of tremor seen in Parkinsonian patients (present at rest, disappearing on voluntary action).

He suggested the name of '*sclerose en plaques*', by which he meant hardening '*sclerose*' or scarring in the nervous system due to the disease process. As many physicians are today, he was worried about this name and its implications to patients, relatives and doctors alike. One group of symptoms seen in multiple sclerosis is still called 'Charcot's triad', namely, nystagmus, intention tremor and scanning speech (see chapter 5).

Defining multiple sclerosis

Multiple sclerosis can be defined as 'a disease of unknown aetiology, characterised pathologically by the widespread occurrence in the nervous system of patches of demyelination followed by gliosis'. (Walton, 1977). To this it must be added that relapses and remissions are a striking feature of this disease, which may be prolonged for many years. A different way of defining multiple sclerosis is to examine the individual characteristics of the disease. This method provides a data base for any individual patient (Capildeo *et al.*, 1980).

Age at presentation

Multiple sclerosis presenting before the age of 10 years and after the age of 50 is exceedingly rare. This means that the diagnosis should be questioned in any patient presenting for the first time outside this age limit. In older patients, a careful history may indicate that the symptoms of the disease started many years before diagnosis (see chapter 9).

History

The most important feature of this disease is the history of relapses and remissions. This implies that after one attack a definite diagnosis cannot be made, although the 'attack' itself may be typical. This classical approach to the diagnosis of multiple sclerosis has changed because of the introduction of new neurophysiological tests and improved alternative methods for the examination of cerebrospinal fluid. However, caution should be taken regarding the early diagnosis of multiple sclerosis after the history of only one attack. A progressive history must be substantiated by clinical findings and investigations before the diagnosis of multiple sclerosis is made.

Clinical findings

One of the commonest modes of presentation is *optic neuritis*, that is, acute pain in one eye on movement, acute loss of vision and swelling of the optic disc on ophthalmoscopy. In the UK, the only cause for acute optic neuritis in a young person is acute demyelination, but only about one-third of patients will go on to have further attacks.

Weakness and spasticity of both legs (*spastic paraparesis*) is also a common presentation, indicating upper motor neurone involvement. The usual site of the lesion is in the *cervical cord*.

The presence of *nystagmus*, particularly when associated with an internuclear ophthalmoplegia (so that the eyes do not move conjugately) indicates a lesion in the *brainstem*.

Intention tremor and *ataxia* of the legs indicate *cerebellar involvement*.

Dysarthria, sensory symptoms and *incontinence* are also common. Rarely, motor weakness may first affect a single limb or even cause a hemiparesis. The pattern of the clinical signs will indicate dissemination of lesions throughout the central nervous system, for example, emotional lability (frontal lobes), optic neuritis (optic nerve), nystagmus (brainstem), intention tremor and ataxia (cerebellum), spastic paraparesis (cervical cord).

The diagnosis of multiple sclerosis is 'clinically definite' if (a) the symptoms and signs have been present for more than one year, (b) the patient has had several episodes with remissions, and (c) the clinical signs indicate two or more lesions in the central nervous system. A proven diagnosis is, strictly speaking, reserved for cases in which there has been confirmation by autopsy.

Investigations

There is no definite diagnostic test for multiple sclerosis. Fields *et al.* (1974), initially using a lymphocyte migration test, thought that they had a definite test for multiple sclerosis. Unfortunately this test has not been confirmed by other workers. Using red blood cells from multiple sclerosis patients, positive results have been claimed by Zukoski *et al.* (1979) from Portland, Oregon. In the test, red blood cells are exposed to an electric field and the mobility of the cells can be affected by the addition of linoleic and arachidonic acids (polyunsaturated fats, see chapter 7). The cells from multiple sclerosis patients slow down whilst those from normal patients speed up.

At Charing Cross Hospital, we are attempting to repeat this test and the results look promising (Jones *et al.*, 1981). It will have important implications if positive. The test could then be used to detect patients with early disease, people at risk and even people who might react positively and yet not have the disease. If susceptibility to multiple sclerosis is determined genetically, then the pattern of inheritance might also be determined.

At the moment, other practical tests are available which help to confirm the presence of optic nerve lesions and also brainstem lesions. Demyelination in the optic nerve will cause delay in the transmission of impulses from the retina to the visual area in the occipital cortex. The time can be measured neurophysiologically and is known as the *visual evoked response* (VER)*. The subject looks either at a flashing light or at a chequerboard pattern which produces an alternating signal (the black and white squares alternate one square every second) and the average of several hundred stimuli (usually 250) are recorded by means of electroencephalographic leads placed over the occiput. The time taken (in milliseconds) for the signal to be relayed to the occipital area from the retina is therefore measured. A characteristic normal wave form indi-

*Also called VEP (visual evoked potential).

cates a large negative depression at about 100 milliseconds. In patients with optic neuritis, this is delayed, either in one eye, so that there is an intra-ocular difference, or in both eyes, often up to 140 milliseconds.

The importance of the test is that in most patients it remains abnormal even when the optic neuritis recovers clinically with full restoration of vision. In other patients, who give no history of optic neuritis, the VERs may also be delayed. The VERs are abnormal in about 70 per cent of multiple sclerosis patients. Therefore, the test can be used to detect an otherwise unsuspected central nervous system lesion which may make the diagnosis of multiple sclerosis likely even when there is only a short history, or a history of one clinical episode. If the patient is 30 years old and presents with an acute onset of spastic paraparesis, abnormal VERs would mean that a second lesion was also present. Patients who have exhibited one clinical episode and at least two separate central nervous system lesions are often said to have 'early probable' or 'latent' multiple sclerosis.

Two other neurophysiological tests may be performed but are probably less useful. The *auditory evoked responses* can be measured in a similar way using a repetitive auditory click. A delay will usually indicate brainstem involvement, although delay could occur anywhere along the auditory sensory pathway. The test is abnormal in about 30 per cent of clinically definite cases of multiple sclerosis. Sensory evoked potentials, stimulating one arm, produce responses in the neck and over the scalp which depend upon conduction along the sensory pathways passing from the spinal cord to the brain. These tests may confirm clinical findings, and in the case of VERs they may detect unsuspected lesions.

Examination of the *cerebrospinal fluid* may indicate an increase in the number of lymphocytes during a relapse. There may also be a rise in the protein, mainly an excess of globulin. Immunoelectrophoresis of the globulin fraction may show the presence of oligoclonal bands. This test is positive in less than 70 per cent of multiple sclerosis patients.

Computerised axial tomography (CAT scanning) may demonstrate plaques, particularly around the ventricles. Further evolution of this technique may help to detect plaques more easily than is possible at present.

The value of these tests is that they may confirm our clinical diagnosis and eventually, as further tests are developed, a definite test may be found. If a patient has 'clinically definitive' multiple sclerosis, with abnormal VERs and oligoclonal bands in the cerebrospinal fluid, then the diagnosis is confirmed as far as possible. If the VERs in this patient are normal (when the patient has 'clinically definitive' multiple sclerosis, the likelihood is greater than 90 per cent that the VERs will be abnormal), as is the cerebrospinal fluid examination, then the diagnosis would be open to doubt. It is possible that this patient may be quite different from the 'typical' case, although both patients may subsequently be proved to have multiple sclerosis.

Other factors

Sex

Multiple sclerosis occurs more frequently in females, but this factor is not of diagnostic importance.

Geography

Multiple sclerosis is very common in temperate zones. A background knowledge of our patients will determine whether the patient has lived in a high risk area at a crucial age (see page 10).

Race

Multiple sclerosis is less common in some races (e.g. Indians and black South Africans). However, if a person is born and lives in a high risk area then this factor appears to outweigh any genetic factor which might otherwise be protective.

Heredity

It has been estimated that the risk of developing multiple sclerosis is 15 times greater in a first degree relative, and two siblings may both be affected. The involvement of two generations is less common. Epidemiological studies (page 10) suggest that there is a critical period when the disease may be acquired. The evidence that certain of the histocompatability antigens (HLA 3 and 7, DW2) are more common in multiple sclerosis patients has not been proven when compared with control subjects from the general population.

In Summary

Multiple sclerosis can be defined on the basis of history, clinical examination and investigations, that is, *age at presentation, a history of relapses and remissions, the duration of the disease being greater than one year, the presence of lesions scattered in the central nervous system as indicated by the clinical signs and confirmatory investigations.*

Anatomical and pathological features

The anatomical feature of multiple sclerosis is that the lesions are confined to the central nervous system, that is, the brain and spinal cord. The peripheral nerves are not involved.

The pathological feature of multiple sclerosis is the plaques. As yet it is not certain whether myelin is damaged first or whether the first change is the collection of lymphocytes around small perforating veins in the central nervous system. Degeneration of myelin leads to the formation of the plaques, which become swollen. Rapid improvement after an acute attack of multiple sclerosis is due to the resolution of oedema and improved conduction down the axon. The severity of the lesion depends on the size of each plaque, the degree of activity of the plaque, for example, extension of the plaque due to continued activity of lymphocytes at the perimeter of the plaque, and the degree of axonal damage. Fortunately, axons remain intact unless the disease is very advanced. It is not yet certain whether re-myelination occurs in the central nervous system. Particular sites of predilection for plaque formation are the optic nerve and cervical cord.

Epidemiological studies

Epidemiological studies have provided important clues to the aetiology of multiple sclerosis. Prevalence rates (the number of cases in every 100 000 of the population with the disease as measured on a specific day) have been measured in a number of countries. In the United Kingdom, the prevalence rate is 50 per 100 000, but there are regional variations. Some of the highest rates ever reported are to be found in north-eastern Scotland (100 per 100 000) and on the Orkney and Shetland Islands (100–300 per 100 000). In the United States of America, rates are four times higher in the northern states of America than in the southern states.

Kurtzke (1980*a*) defines a high frequency zone with a prevalence of at least 30–80 per 100 000 extending from 43° to 65° north latitude and a medium frequency zone from about 38° to 46°, with rates of between 5 and 25 per 100 000, and most within the range 10–15 per 100 000. Intermediate zones include the southern states of America, northern Australia, and the Mediterranean. Although Japan is in the high frequency zone according to latitude, multiple sclerosis is rare.

In South Africa, multiple sclerosis does occur in the white population, although rare, and is virtually absent in the black population. In the United States of America, the prevalence rates closely approximate between the white and black population. Multiple sclerosis is unknown among Eskimos. In the Faroe Islands, the increased prevalence of multiple sclerosis since 1949 has been put down to the fact that British troops (mostly Scottish) were based there during the Second World War (Kurtzke, 1980*b*). Migration studies have indicated that the risk of getting multiple sclerosis remains high if a person moves from a high risk area over to a low risk area after the age of 15 years. More recently, it has been suggested that the critical age may be up to 5 years of age. Europeans, particularly of Scandinavian stock, appear to be most susceptible to multiple sclerosis. In general, multiple sclerosis is more common in rural than urban areas.

Theories of causation

From the results of these studies, it has been suggested that multiple sclerosis is due to a 'slow virus' infection, the virus being contracted by the age of 15 years, lying dormant, to become active many years later. The trigger that activates the virus is not known. The geographic variation would favour a viral hypothesis, but the virus that has received most attention, the measles virus, is world-wide. So if multiple sclerosis is due to a slow virus, is the virus one that is already well known to us or is it a new virus? Migration studies suggest that moving into high risk areas at a certain age increases the risk; in other words, geographical factors may be more important than racial characteristics or genetic background. However, susceptibility may depend upon the genetic makeup. Is the virus like the cold sore virus, herpes simplex? Herpes simplex is very common, yet only in some people does it cause cold sores, whilst in others it may cause encephalitis. It is implicated in cancer of the cervix. People who get cold sores generally feel 'run down' a day or two before the cold sore appears. Feeling 'run down' probably has an immunological basis, but as yet we have no way of measuring this. The herpes simplex virus lives in the mouth. Like the shingles virus, herpes zoster, it may be present for many years before it becomes apparent. It is well known that herpes zoster can cause chickenpox in children and shingles in 'Grandma'. If the virus is present in the body, then relapses and remissions cannot be the explanation for infection or reinfection. The individual's body response to the virus would be more likely to determine whether the person has a mild or progressive illness.

The role of diet may be important (see chapter 7) and environmental factors must also be considered. Controlling all these variables makes multiple sclerosis research extraordinarily difficult. One approach is to study family groups with two or more affected individuals. In addition to studying people who have multiple sclerosis, it is important to study control subjects from the normal population in an attempt to determine why they have *not* got the disease. The study of poliomyelitis is a good example of this approach. (Children of higher social classes were less likely to come into contact with poliomyelitis than children from more socially deprived backgrounds. When the epidemic occurred, the children from the lower social classes were more likely to be protected because of antibodies formed during a subclinical infection.)

Another intriguing group of subjects that it might be possible to designate if a diagnostic blood test becomes available would be those who might have 'the virus' but who do not develop multiple sclerosis (as opposed to those subjects who are positive and do develop the disease).

A recent hypothesis (Martin, 1981) suggests that herpes simplex may be the aetiological agent. There are two known types of herpes simplex virus: HSV-1 and HSV-2. The theory is that HSV-1 may provide immunity from subsequent infection by HSV-2; therefore people lacking HSV-1 immunity may be at risk from HSV-2 infection, which might then cause multiple sclerosis.

Prognosis

Unfortunately, the popular concept of multiple sclerosis is that all patients will end up in a wheel-chair. In fact, less than 10 per cent of patients with multiple sclerosis will require wheel-chair care. In hospital, our view of multiple sclerosis is distorted since we tend to see acute patients and the most severely affected individuals. Optic neuritis (or retrobulbar neuritis) has a good prognosis; many years may pass before there is a further attack. Up to 20 years is not unusual. Very rarely an acute attack of multiple sclerosis may be fatal. Many patients lead a normal life with minimal disability, and the general rule is that patients recover from an acute attack. About one-third may have residual disability afterwards and further disability may accrue with further attacks (see page 10, chapter 9).

The patients with a poor prognosis are those with a progressive history, often over a 3 year period, who also have severe cerebellar ataxia. Variability on a day to day basis, often associated with fatigue or sensory phenomena, is very difficult to interpret. Some patients find it difficult to recount definite relapses. In other patients, it is difficult to believe how severe an initial episode was when reviewing the patient many months later. Hence, prognosis should always be guarded but can usually be optimistic. This is only justified if the patient is followed up on a regular basis.

Treatment

Accurate detailed assessment of the patient (by the rehabilitation team) in hospital and at home is essential before any type of treatment is complemented. A social network diagram may be a useful visual aid (Capildeo *et al.*, 1976) (see appendix to chapter 4, page 58).

As yet there is no known cure for multiple sclerosis. Steroids, Prednisolone or ACTH are often used, yet no clear benefit has been demonstrated by properly controlled clinical trials. Patients who have disturbances of affect may be helped. High dose steroids have yet to be fully assessed but seem promising. Vitamin B injections, particularly vitamin B12, are often prescribed, but the evidence of benefit is inconclusive. Diet is considered in chapter 7. Drugs to reduce spasticity may be very helpful to the patient, such as Lioresal and Dantrolene sodium. These drugs must be titrated according to the patient's requirements. Incontinence may prove a serious problem. Treatment is considered in chapter 2. Rehabilitation in the context of the rehabilitation team is the main aim of treatment and is separately considered in each of the subsequent chapters.

Further controlled clinical trials are essential, particularly to determine whether immunosuppression or enhancement is an important factor. Until the aetiology of multiple sclerosis is determined, treatment will continue to be empirical.

Summary

In this chapter, the current medical status of multiple sclerosis has been reviewed in order to provide a background for the further chapters in this book. There is no room for pessimism in this disease. Research into multiple sclerosis has reached an exciting stage.

From our follow-up of a large number of patients, at home and attending hospital clinics, it is quite clear that the majority of patients have mild to moderate disability and that most are helped by the rehabilitation team. Education is of prime importance - to keep the individual patient, caring relatives and friends up to date as well as the rehabilitation team. Involvement in their disease through one of the voluntary societies (chapter 8) also adds a new dimension to their lives.

References

Capildeo, R. (1982). Charcot in the '80's'. In *Historical Aspects of the Neurosciences* (Ed. W. Bynum and F. Clifford Rose), Raven Press, New York.

Capildeo, R., Court, C. and Rose, F. C. (1976). Social network diagram. *Br. med. J.* 1, 143-4.

Capildeo, R., Haberman, S. and Rose, F. C. (1980). The classification and coding of neurological disease. In *Clinical Neuroepidemiology* (Ed. F. Clifford Rose), Pitman Medical, Tunbridge Wells.

Fields, E. J., Shenton, B. K. and Joyce, G. (1974). Specific laboratory test for the diagnosis of multiple sclerosis. *Br. med. J.* 1, 412-4.

Jones, R., Capildeo, R., Luckman, N. P., Preece, A. W., Forrester, J. A. and Rose, F. C. (1981). A diagnostic test for multiple sclerosis using glutaraldehyde fixed erythrocytes and laser cytophotometry. In *Cell Electrophoresis in Cancer and other Clinical Research* (Ed. A. W. Preece and P. A. Light), Elsevier-North Holland Biomedical Press.

Kurtzke, J. (1980*a*). Multiple sclerosis: an overview. In *Clinical Neuroepidemiology* (Ed. F. Clifford Rose), Pitman Medical, Tunbridge Wells.

Kurtzke, J. (1980*b*). Multiple sclerosis in the Faroe Islands. In *Clinical Neuroepidemiology* (Ed. F. Clifford Rose), Pitman Medical, Tunbridge Wells.

Martin, J. (1981). Herpes simplex virus types 1 and 2 and multiple sclerosis. *Lancet, ii*, 777-81.

Walton, J. (1977). *Brain's Diseases of the Nervous System*, 8th edn, Oxford University Press.

Zukoski, C. F., Tamblyn, C. H., Swank, R. L. and Seaman, G. V. F. (1979). The basis for the unsaturated fatty acid red cell electrophoretic mobility test for multiple sclerosis. In *Cell Electrophoresis: Clinical Application and Methodology* (Ed. A. W. Preece and D. Sabolovic), Elsevier-North Holland Biomedical Press.

2 Surgical aspects of multiple sclerosis

C. H. Hawkes, R. Beard and D. G. Thomas

Contrary to expectation the use of surgery in multiple sclerosis is an extensive topic, but many of the surgical options available are 'last resort' measures - few offer real value in terms of alteration of a patient's way of life.

Should a patient with multiple sclerosis have an operation at all? This question was considered by Ridley and Schapira (1961) when they studied 662 patients with multiple sclerosis, 40 of whom had 57 operations under general anaesthesia. Although surgery was followed by no acute relapse, eight patients gradually deteriorated within one month of operation, giving an overall risk of 14 per cent. Hence surgery in multiple sclerosis carries a small risk of aggravating the disease, but not sufficient to justify avoidance of a necessary operation.

Surgical aspects of multiple sclerosis may be discussed under the following headings: (a) tremor, (b) pain, (c) spasticity, (d) impotence, (e) bladder disorder.

Tremor

Cerebellar tremor, characterised by rapid movements of the limb, usually on voluntary movement, relieved by rest, can be particularly disabling and if severe and bilateral - even in the absence of weakness - is tantamount to paralysis.

There are currently no drugs suitable for cerebellar tremor and thalamic surgery offers the only hope of relief. Thalamotomy, first used by Cooper (1960), involves a lesion in the medial portion of the ventrolateral nucleus of the contralateral thalamus. In his first six patients, two of whom had multiple sclerosis, uniformly good results were reported.

A more extensive and critical review was presented 10 years later (Samra *et al.*, 1970) in a series of 73 patients, of whom 25 had multiple sclerosis. 'Excellent' relief of tremor was obtained in 13 (multiple sclerosis patients) and 'good' relief in seven; the remaining five cases showed little change. Approximately 10 per cent of the 73 patients experienced confusion, difficulty with balance, dysphasia and dysarthria. Although the complications were stated to be transient and to respond well to physiotherapy or speech therapy, they were more prevalent in the multiple sclerosis patients.

The creation of a further lesion in a usually progressive disease such as multiple sclerosis is clearly undesirable. Hence the thalamic stimulation technique described recently by Brice and McLellan (1980) is particularly attractive. Electrodes are permanently inserted into the thalamo-mesencephalic junctional area, contralateral to the side of tremor. The electrodes are activated only in response to a signal generated from the electromyogram of the deltoid muscle of the affected arm. Because the apparatus only operates when required, the potential dangers of continuous stimulation and possible cell damage are avoided. Brice and McLellan (1980) report complete suppression of tremor in three patients with multiple sclerosis, with maintenance of effect over a 6 month period. Transient deterioration of clinical signs was noted in these patients, of similar nature to those described by Samra *et al.* (1970), but no relapses occurred.

Pain

Trigeminal neuralgia, namely brief paroxysmal attacks of severe pain occurring in the distribution of one or more branches of the trigeminal nerve, brought on by 'triggers' such as washing the face, may rarely be the presenting symptom of multiple sclerosis, but more often it complicates established disease. In character it is identical to idiopathic '*tic douloureux*' experienced by elderly people. It can normally be suppressed by carbamazepine (Tegretol) and/or phenytoin (Epanutin). When drug treatment fails to control the 'tic', or if there are unacceptable side effects of the medical treatment, for example anaemia, skin rash, drowsiness or ataxia, then neurosurgical treatment may be required. Several closed and open procedures are available.

Closed procedures

In most centres selective percutaneous radiofrequency coagulation of the trigeminal ganglion has superseded injection of alcohol or phenol into the ganglion. The radiofrequency coagulation method delivers heat locally from the tip of a probe electrode, the position, length and temperature of which may be accurately controlled to destroy pain-sensitive fibres in mandibular, maxillary or ophthalmic divisions of the trigeminal nerve. Since 'tic' seldom affects the ophthalmic division it is generally possible by this procedure, in contrast to the alcohol injection method, to spare corneal sensation as well as to retain some sensation of touch in the rest of the face. This avoids the principal undesirable complications which may follow alcohol injection, namely profound numbness of the face, anaesthesia dolorosa, and a tendency to develop corneal ulcers.

Open procedures

The trigeminal nerve may be sectioned surgically at any point in its course. Division and avulsion of the peripheral nerve branches in the supraorbital notch, in the infraorbital foramen or in the dental canal may be done relatively simply but is usually of temporary benefit only. Section of the ganglion in Meckel's cave or of the sensory root adjacent to the brainstem in the posterior fossa are more permanent remedies for 'tic', but require major operations. Tractotomy of the descending tract of the trigeminal nerve in the medulla (Sjöqvist's operation) can be performed at open operation or percutaneously by stereotactic methods. However, this procedure carries greater risk and is only indicated after other methods have failed.

Of these various surgical operations available for treatment of trigeminal neuralgia in the patient with multiple sclerosis, the percutaneous radiofrequency coagulation is generally most appropriate.

Late on in the disease patients with multiple sclerosis may experience unusual discomfort called 'central' pain, thought to be due to demyelination in the spinothalamic tracts. The pain is typically continuous, diffuse and burning, usually felt over the legs or trunk and refractory to all analgesia apart from opiates. Such pain may occasionally respond to stellate ganglion block (Loh *et al.*, 1981), transcutaneous nerve stimulation (Bates, 1981) or dorsal column stimulation (Hawkes *et al.*, 1980).

Spasticity

Frequent flexor or extensor spasms, severe spasticity and contractures in multiple sclerosis are largely things of the past with the advent of skilled physiotherapy and two potent antispastic drugs, baclofen (Lioresal) and dantrolene (Dantrium). Formerly, surgical measures such as tenotomy, neurectomy or rhizotomy were needed to enable passive movement of the limb and facilitate nursing. Intrathecal phenol first introduced by Nathan (1965) was used in refractory cases with good effect. The procedure still has a limited place in relief of spasticity but because bladder fibres may be damaged it is contraindicated if the patient is continent.

There are many devices available which stimulate peripheral nerve or muscle directly. These include the relatively simple portable apparatus for spastic wrist or foot drop and highly complex multi-electrode microprocessor-controlled muscle stimulators which have been used in hemiplegic lower limbs. All these appliances are still in the developmental stage but are the subject of considerable research activity, largely outside the United Kingdom (Trnkoczy *et al.*, 1978). It is likely that patients with hemiplegia will be the first to benefit from such advances. The multiple sclerosis patient with paraplegia will have to wait longer because the electronic problems associated with co-ordination of two limbs are formidable. Nevertheless, it is quite conceivable that patients with paraplegia from multiple sclerosis or from spinal trauma could be restored to walking by functional electrical stimulation in the not too distant future.

Chronic cerebellar stimulation has been used in the management of spasticity, in particular in cases of cerebral palsy. According to Cooper *et al.*, (1976) striking benefit in terms of muscle tone and mobility may be gained from this procedure: however, his patients all received physiotherapy and it is impossible to know which technique produced the improvement so claimed. A double-blind cross-over trial by Gahm *et al.* (1981) in eight patients suggested that the procedure has no influence on spasticity.

It has been claimed that dorsal column stimulation will help limb spasticity (Cook and Weinstein, 1973; Read *et al.*, 1980) and indeed the studies of Illis *et al.* (1976) on 'H' reflex excitability curves (which indirectly measure spasticity) suggested a real effect. Hawkes *et al.* (1980), in a detailed assessment by clinical evaluation, timed tasks and videotape recordings, found no evidence of improved muscle tone. The issue is, as yet, unresolved, but whatever the outcome it matters little as the effects are only slight and can readily be produced by antispastic drugs mentioned above.

Impotence

Impotence is common in multiple sclerosis, and may be the basis of further domestic problems. Sympathetic counselling, if required, can be arranged through Sexual Problems of the Disabled (SPOD; Telephone 01 486 9823). Surgery is available only in the form of implantable silicone penile prosthesis, thereby making penetration possible. There are three varieties of implant available: rigid, hinged/flexible and inflatable. The last type, that designed by Scott *et al.* (1973) and supplied by American Medical Systems Inc., is the most functionally realistic but not without its drawbacks - cost, complexity, need for manual dexterity, and long term mechanical failure.

Recently Brindley (1981) has shown that it is feasible to induce ejaculation electrically by rectal stimulation. The majority of his 84 patients had spinal injury and he was able to obtain semen from the majority. Its effect in multiple sclerosis is not discussed, but there is no theoretical reason why equally good results should not be achieved.

Bladder disorder

It is estimated that 80 per cent of patients with multiple sclerosis have bladder symptoms at some stage of the disease. However, in approximately 2–5 per cent, the first symptoms of the disease are urinary. Several factors make the urological management of the patient difficult. First, the clinical course of the disease is very variable but usually progressive. Secondly, urological symptoms correlate poorly with the underlying urodynamic abnormality; furthermore, the urodynamic findings may change with time. Thirdly, there is no satisfactory external urinary appliance available for women.

In general terms, urodynamic assessment may demonstrate that the bladder muscle (detrusor) is hyperactive, that is, it responds to filling by an uninhibited contraction, or more rarely is atonic when no evidence of detrusor activity can be elicited. In addition it is possible to assess the outflow resistance and, in particular, to document the failure of the urethral sphincter to relax during micturition (urethral sphincter dyssynergia). Continence depends on the outflow (urethral) resistance being greater than the intravesical pressure at all times except during voluntary micturition. Conversely, the ability of the bladder to empty depends on the pressure generated in the bladder to be greater, throughout micturition, than the outflow resistance. In managing these patients the clinician's aim should be to preserve renal function by correcting any obstruction and by eliminating or at least greatly reducing infection.

In addition the patient should be made continent or, failing this, dry. In practice this is often a compromise. It is also important that the facilities at home are usable by the disabled patient. Having assessed the renal function, the state of the upper tracts, and the presence of infection, several options are available. The detrusor hyperactivity may be reduced by anticholinergic drugs such as emepronium bromide (Cetiprin) and propantheline bromide (ProBanthine) or by hydrostatic dilatation of the bladder. In practice these manoeuvres are really of benefit only in mild cases. The urethral resistance can be lowered by an α-adrenergic blocker such as phenoxybenzamine, by urethral dilation or by urethrotomy. If there is upper tract dilatation on the intravenous urogram (IVU), which only occurs in male patients, this should ideally be corrected even at the price of rendering the patient incontinent. This may be achieved by division of the external sphincter transurethrally plus resecting the prostate if necessary. The majority of such male patients can be made dry using a condom appliance and a leg bag. On occasions this is not possible, due to small penis size or penile ulceration from the appliance. In these patients the only alternatives are long term silastic catheter drainage or urinary diversion into an ileal loop.

Female patients often pose a difficult problem of recurrent infection, incomplete emptying and urge incontinence. If the incontinence cannot be controlled by drugs or hydrostatic dilation, the choice lies between urethral catheterisation and some form of urinary diversion. The latter is probably best achieved by constructing an ileal conduit, after which the patient wears a collecting bag over a stoma on the abdominal wall. Although this is a relatively major operation, the results in terms of renal preservation and patient acceptance are satisfactory. The only real contraindication to major surgery of this kind is the presence of pressure sores (Desmond and Shuttleworth, 1977).

It should be stressed that the reason diversion is so commonly undertaken in such disabled patients is that there is often no other way of diminishing the power and frequency of the uninhibited detrusor contractions (UDC). These contractions may cause incontinence even in catheterised women. Recently considerable success has been achieved in abolishing UDC by endoscopically injecting phenol deep to the base of the bladder. Although this study is in its infancy the results so far are encouraging (Beard and Shuttleworth, 1981).

In assessing the value of any treatment it should be emphasised that a small improvement in bladder control may be greatly appreciated in women for whom the alternative is a catheter or diversion. In men small gains of bladder control are not so valued, as the condom appliance with or without sphincter and/or prostatic surgery is simple and convenient.

In summary, there are only two widely available surgical options for the patient with severe bladder dysfunction: (a) in men, sphincter destruction and the use of a condom appliance; (b) in women, diversion by means of an ileal conduit.

There is a variety of electrical means by which a spastic bladder may be improved, which at present are at the experimental stage:

(a) *Direct detrusor stimulation*. In this the bladder is stimulated directly by means of implanted electrodes. According to Merrill (1976), 50 per cent of patients benefited from this, but in general the technique has found little favour elsewhere and had been abandoned.

(b) *Conus medullaris implant*. Electrodes are inserted directly into the conus medullaris, and activated by radiofrequency coupling (Nashold *et al*., 1977). In their report of 11 traumatic paraplegics, eight regained control of voiding. There are no reports of its use in multiple sclerosis, and the technique does not benefit dyssynergia.

(c) *Sacral anterior root stimulation* (Brindley, 1977). This ingenious technique utilises electrodes implanted on the sacral anterior (motor) roots. By careful adjustment of the strength and pattern of stimulation it is possible to contract detrusor or sphincter muscle independently, making the patient continent or allowing him to void at will. This has so far been tried in seven paraplegics with good results; poor results were obtained in one patient with multiple sclerosis (G. S. Brindley, personal communication).

We conclude this section on surgical improvement of bladder disorder with a review of dorsal column stimulation (DCS) in multiple sclerosis. Although there are claims of wide ranging benefit in the disease, there is almost universal agreement that the chief effect of DCS is on bladder dysfunction.

Dorsal column stimulation (DCS)

This procedure has a small but established place in the management of refractory pain. In 1973 Cook happened to treat a patient for pain secondary to multiple sclerosis and discovered that not only was pain relieved but the patient could, for the first time, lift her legs (Cook, 1976). This chance observation has led to numerous reports, mostly anecdotal or uncritical, claiming benefit in almost every aspect of the disease.

The technique basically involves placement of one or two electrodes in the epidural space over the midline, typically at mid-thoracic level. Electrodes may be inserted percutaneously or by laminectomy. Stimulation comes from a pocket-sized battery-powered multivibrator which transmits via an antenna through the skin to a receiving coil embedded in the subcutaneous tissue of the trunk. The epidural electrodes are activated by the receiving coil, which characteristically delivers a signal of 33 Hz, 200 ms pulse width and 6–12 V. The output is adjusted so that the patient just begins to feel a tingling sensation, normally in the lower limbs.

In our first survey of 19 patients so treated (Hawkes *et al.*, 1980) we found no convincing evidence of improvement over a two week period in any aspect of voluntary motor function or sensation. However, many patients considered that they had improved (chiefly in walking) and, despite the fact that formal physiotherapy was not permitted, exercised themselves frequently! When allowance was made for this and the inevitably high motivation in many individuals, no genuine change was though to have occurred. Slight gains in hip flexor power and grip strength were sometimes seen, but these muscles can readily be improved by simple training (Tourtelotte *et al.*, 1965). Similar observations in motor function were made by Read *et al.* (1980), although on the basis of clinical examination they felt that spasticity was lessened.

The authors do not feel that this issue is resolved as yet. No one has measured spasticity in DCS by other than bedside techniques, which are at best crude. Multiple sclerosis is an illness whose symptoms and signs may vary considerably from day to day or from hour to hour even in apparent remission. The detection of a real effect of treatment against this background 'noise' is formidable and can probably only be achieved by multiple observation and statistical examination.

In studies of bladder response to DCS over the past three

years, a total of 26 patients with definite, clinically stable multiple sclerosis have been examined (Hawkes *et al.*, 1981). The stimulation technique involved two epidural electrodes positioned 2–3 cm apart in the mid-thoracic vertebral area. Patients were assessed on two occasions prior to DCS and then twice during the two weeks of continuous stimulation. Assessment consisted of the following:

(a) *Documentation of urinary output* (volume and time taken). Initially this was performed manually but subsequently (nine patients) was carried out electronically, using a DISA mictiograph. The latter allowed the urinary flow pattern and peak flow rate to be measured.

(b) *Cine cystometrogram.*

(c) *Urethral pressure profile studies.* Effect of α-adrenergic blockade with phentolamine.

The majority of patients (73 per cent) reported improvement in urinary stream and about half noted lessening of urgency. Improvement in continence was least often observed.

The urodynamic changes were assessed on an arbitrary basis using a three-point scale following discussion between the two leading authors. This was necessary because of the small numbers involved. There was no change in the residual urine estimation, and in approximately half of the patients (six out of 13) there appeared to be a delay in the onset of the uninhibited detrusor contractions. The urethral pressure profiles were examined statistically and no changes were found following DCS. Although not significant, it did appear that the fall in urethral closing pressure which occurs after intravenous phentolamine (an α-adrenergic blocker) was not so marked when the DCS was in progress.

The data obtained from urinary flow analysis using the mictiograph showed significant (matched pair 't' test $p = 0.05$) improvement in one or more aspects of flow in five of the nine subjects examined. Parameters most frequently improved were peak flow and hesitancy. Ten previous patients (Hawkes *et al.*, 1980) were also examined statistically, but only data for volume and voiding times were available – not flow patterns. Combining these results, improvement in one or more parameters was seen in 14 out of 19 subjects; two were worse;

three were unaltered. Mean or peak flow changes were seen most often. By combining urinary flow data in 10 patients who showed clear improvement it was found that the bladder response to DCS gradually increased and then stabilised at day 6 or day 7. Return to basal values was found to be slow if the stimulation ceased; such return was the more gradual the longer stimulation had been in progress.

We considered that DCS was producing a genuine improvement in the urinary flow rates. The mechanism by which it occurs is less clear, but our results suggest that there is a reduction in that component of the outflow resistance, which is due to α-adrenergic activity.

The majority of other workers on DCS (Cook and Weinstein, 1973; Illis *et al.*, 1980; Read *et al.*, 1980) have found improvement in bladder function along broadly similar lines. Some have claimed improvement in continence and even abandonment of an indwelling catheter (Illis *et al.*, 1980), but these claims have never been supported by detailed urodynamic and flow studies.

We feel that DCS has been shown to have a small beneficial effect on bladder function in carefully selected patients. The procedure is time-consuming both to doctor and patient, and electronic failure is common. Three of our patients – all in an originally stable condition – had minor relapses during or shortly after the stimulation period. We were only able to alter the patients' 'way of life' to a mild degree, and one must seriously question whether the time and expense is worthwhile. We feel that DCS is still an experimental procedure which cannot be generally recommended at present. Improvement of electrode design and drastic lowering of cost in the future is badly needed.

Acknowledgements

The authors would like to acknowledge the kind assistance of Professor W. I. McDonald, Institute of Neurology, Queen Square, London, and Mr K. E. D. Shuttleworth, Department of Urology, St Thomas' Hospital, London, for advice in compiling this review.

References

Bates, J. A. V. (1978). Therapeutic electrical stimulation. The transistorized placebo? In *Contemporary Clinical Neurophysiology* (Ed. W. A. Cobb and H. Van Duijn), EEG Supplement No. 34, pp. 329-34.

Beard, R. and Shuttleworth, K. E. (1981). The abolition of uninhibited detrusor contractions in patients with multiple sclerosis by subtrigonal injection of phenol. In preparation.

Brice, J. and McLellan, L. (1980). Suppression of intention tremor by contingent deep-brain stimulation. *Lancet i*, 1221-2.

Brindley, G. S. (1977). An implant to empty the bladder or close the uretha. *J. Neurol. Neurosurg. Psychiat.* 40, 358-69.

Brindley, G. S. (1981). Electroejaculation: its technique, neurological implications and uses. *J. Neurol. Neurosurg. Psychiat.* 44, 9-18.

Cook, A. W. (1976). Electrical stimulation in multiple sclerosis. *Hospital Practice* 2, 51-8.

Cook, A. W. and Weinstein, S. P. (1973). Chronic dorsal column stimulation in multiple sclerosis. *N. Y. State J. Med.* 73, 2868-72.

Cooper, I. S. (1960). Neurosurgical relief of intention tremor due to cerebellar disease and multiple sclerosis. *Arch. phys. Med.* 41, 1-4.

Cooper, I. S., Riklan, M., Amin, I. and Waltz, J. M. (1976). Chronic cerebellar stimulation in cerebral palsy. *Neurology* 26, 744-53.

Desmond, A. and Shuttleworth, K. E. (1977). Results of urinary diversion in multiple sclerosis. *Br. J. Urol.* 49, 495-502.

Gahm, N. H., Russman, B. S., Cerciello, R. L., Fiorentino, M. R. and McGrath, D. M. (1981). Chronic cerebellar stimulation for cerebral palsy. A double blind study. *Neurology, Minneap.* 31, 87-90.

Hawkes, C. H., Wyke, M., Desmond, A., Bultitude, M. I. and Kanegaonkar, G. S. (1980). Stimulation of dorsal column in multiple sclerosis. *Br. Med. J.* 280, 889-91.

Hawkes, C. H., Fawcett, D., Cooke, E. D., Emson, P. C., Paul, E. A. and Bowcock, S. A. (1981). Dorsal column stimulation in multiple sclerosis: effects on bladder, leg blood flow and peptides. *Appl. Neurophysiol.* (in press).

Illis, L. S., Oygar, A. E., Sedgwick, E. M. and Sabbahi Awadalla, M. A. (1976). Dorsal column stimulation in the rehabilitation of patients with multiple sclerosis. *Lancet i*, 1383-6.

Illis, L. S., Sedgwick, E. M. and Tallis, R. C. (1980). Spinal cord stimulation in multiple sclerosis: clinical results. *J. Neurol. Neurosurg. Psychiat.* 43, 1-14.

Loh, L., Nathan, P. W. and Schott, G. D. (1981). Pain due to lesions of central nervous system removed by sympathetic block. *Br. Med. J.* 282, 1026-8.

Merrill, D. C. (1976). Electric stimulation of the neurogenic bladder (detrusor). Paper presented to the International Symposium on Electric Stimulation of the Neurogenic Bladder, Frankfurt, 5-6 March 1976.

Nashold, B. S., Grimes, J., Friedman, H., Semans, J. and Avery, R. (1977). Electrical stimulation of conus medullaris in the paraplegic. *Appl. Neurophysiol.* 40, 192-207.

Nathan, P. W. (1965). Chemical rhizotomy for relief of spasticity in ambulant patients. *Br. med. J. i*, 1096-100.

Read, D. J., Mathews, W. B. and Higson, R. H. (1980). The effect of spinal cord stimulation on function in patients with multiple sclerosis. *Brain* 103, 803-33.

Ridley, A. and Schapira, K. (1961). Influence of surgical procedures on the course of multiple sclerosis. *Neurology* 11, 81-2.

Samra, K., Waltz, J. M., Riklan, M. Koslow, M. and Cooper, I. S. (1970). Relief of tremor by thalamic surgery. *J. Neurol. Neurosurg. Psychiat.* 33, 7-15.

Scott, F. B., Bradley, W. E. and Timm, G. W. (1973). Management of erectile impotence. Use of implantable inflatable prosthesis. *Urology* 2, 80-2.

Tourtellotte, W. W., Haerer, A. F., Simpson, J. F., Kuzma, J. W. and Sikorski, J. (1965). Quantitative clinical neurological testing. *Ann. N.Y. Acad. Sci.* 122, 480-505.

Trnkoczy, A., Stanic, U. and Malezic, M. (1978). Present state and prospects in the design of multi channel FES stimulators for gait correction in paretic patients. *Tower Int. technomed. Inst. J. Life Sci.* 8, 17-27.

3 Physiotherapy in the management of multiple sclerosis

Jennifer Todd

Principles of physiotherapy are concerned with psychological and with neurological mechanisms, but whatever treatment techniques are introduced or applied it is vital that certain physical management should be given precedence.

Since multiple sclerosis may cause damage anywhere in the brain or spinal cord, the clinical picture is extremely variable. For this reason, it is more important to discuss general principles and guidelines for physiotherapy assessment and treatment than to try to assess different techniques in which benefit has yet to be proven.

These general principles will be discussed under five headings: (a) general philosophy; (b) early advice; (c) maintaining mobility; (d) provision of aids; (e) wheel-chair use.

General philosophy

Therapists pride themselves on individual approaches, yet they are in remarkably constant agreement about overall philosophy.

A positive approach

Most people are aware of the effect of expectation on performance and, because therapists tend to encounter the more severely disabled, care is needed to avoid adopting a pessimistic attitude towards treatment in case it affects outcome. With a positive approach and realistic aims many patients and their families can function adequately and enjoy life in spite of coping with a progressive handicap. They can be encouraged to appreciate a feeling of success at achieving the best level of function possible at each stage of the disease, instead of looking on increasing disability as failure.

It is perhaps easier for some therapists to be more positive if the diagnosis is pushed into the background, and the symptoms are treated as they would if presented with any other form of paralysis.

An integrated team

Integrated management is required because all the specialties overlap and each one requires observations from other areas to provide the most effective care.

Twenty-four hour management

If successful learning and reinforcement is to take place, physical management should not be confined to treatment sessions alone. The manner in which the patient sleeps, sits, moves and performs all the activities in his daily life will affect the level of function. Therefore, without giving full consideration to movement and positioning throughout the 24 hour period, isolated treatment sessions will not be effective. The therapist must allow time to explain – to all concerned – which positions and activities to encourage because they stimulate the required responses and which to avoid because they are likely to be detrimental.

Treatment incorporated into daily life

If suitable activities can be incorporated into the daily routine so that a way of life is established which provides for continuous therapy, the maintenance programme is more likely to be successful.

Prevention

Unfortunately, when a disease is progressive many patients are only referred for physical treatment when they already have established problems. The reason for this may have to do with a misunderstanding of the role of remedial therapy in the general management and in advising about the prevention of secondary handicap. If motor ability is affected, the earlier appropriate management is commenced the more opportunity arises to facilitate potential abilities and to minimise deficits. Therefore good lines of communication with the doctors concerned and other professions working in the community are vital. It is useful if the patient has direct access to the remedial therapy department, because a word of advice given in time can often prevent a problem developing.

Attention to these simple preventative measures will also release valuable treatment time for the more skilled aspects of facilitation of movement.

With increased awareness of the help which can be offered, patients can be treated early enough to prevent the dreadful complications so often accepted as part of the disease.

Responsibility

The prevention of such common problems as pressure sores, contractures and difficulty associated with bladder and bowel dysfunction is comparatively simple, but sometimes insufficient time and care are devoted to initiating or providing a suitable regime which would prevent their occurrence.

The patient must also be encouraged to take responsibility for his own well-being, particularly with regard to skin care, avoidance of contractures, diet, and bladder and bowel function, as we have come to expect from any well trained patient with an injury to the spinal cord.

Early advice

The clinical picture can present a broad spectrum of dysfunction and, in addition to the formidable task of treating the wide variety of possible symptoms, there is the additional difficulty of anticipating complications from the progressive nature of the disease.

The motor disability arises from impairment of the neurological mechanism of *posture*, of *balance* and of *movement*, and although no two people are alike there are certain common features which can be anticipated when any movement deficit is present.

(a) If referred at an early stage, however minor the problem appears to be, a thorough assessment of movement in *all* positions will reveal any imbalance and enable suitable advice to be given to correct any potential lack of symmetry observed.

(b) When appropriate, attention can be given to *activities in daily life* which would stimulate the necessary postural and balance responses.

Example of some activities in daily life which can be so used are as follows:

(a) Head and trunk righting can be stimulated by getting out of bed sideways or when crossing one leg over the other to put on shoes and socks.

(b) Rising reactions are stimulated by standing from sitting without pushing on the hands or by climbing stairs one foot after the other without holding on to the bannister.

(c) Whatever type of abnormal tone is present, loss of trunk rotation and a rounded thoracic spine are typical features which are often overlooked, especially when the deficit is minimal. Adequate stretching will help to prevent this becoming a fixed posture and affecting movement. Suitable activities in which a stretch could be emphasised are (i) reaching for things in cupboards when working in the kitchen or when putting files away in the office and (ii) when dressing by giving an extra stretch each time a shirt or jumper is put on.

(d) The benefits of resting in the prone position can also be introduced at this stage, perhaps when watching television or while reading. A wedge or pillow placed under the chest may help to make it more comfortable.

(e) If the person is advised to continue with the usual occupation and pastimes, and even to take up some form of active sport such as tennis, swimming or riding, the tendency to err on the side of doing too little rather than too much would be avoided.

(f) If adequate adaptation has been made to daily activities it saves devoting time to special exercises and regular out-patient physiotherapy should not be necessary. However, regular follow-up sessions are useful in order to evaluate the programme and to discuss any other problems which arise, or to time refresher courses of intensive therapy to regain lost function. The patient himself may not always notice minor changes which could affect his future prospects.

If the signs change or increase, adjustments in management will be necessary. Advice may be required about diet to control weight or about bladder and bowel management, and the person should fully understand the adverse effects which an inadequate regime will have on abnormal tone and on mobility.

It will probably be appropriate at this stage to give more specific emphasis to the finer control of balance and posture. Additional activities which would stimulate suitable responses can be practised in sitting or standing, using a balance board or a large ball or roll.

Whatever the signs and symptoms, it is possible to anticipate that certain muscle groups tend to become tight unless specific

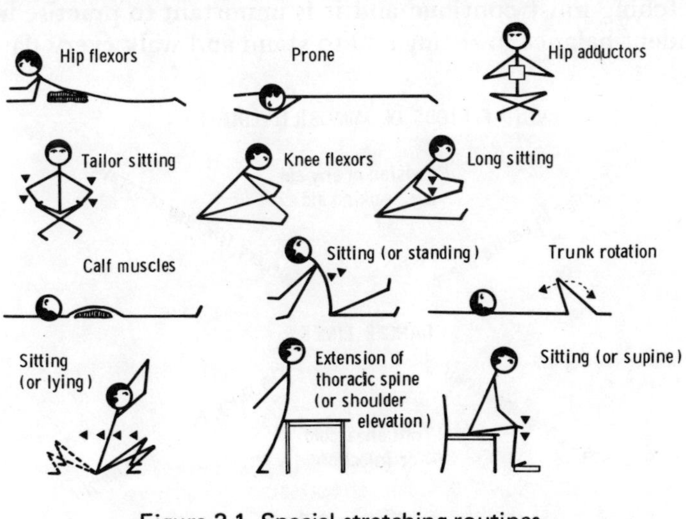

Figure 3.1 Special stretching routines.

stretching techniques are carried out to prevent adaptive shortening. This stretching routine takes a few minutes only, but if carried out daily it provides a simple and certain method of preventing the formation of contractures.

Positions for special stretching exercises are illustrated in figure 3.1 and include the following: (a) hip flexors (prone); (b) hip adductors (tailor sitting); (c) knee flexors (long sitting); (d) calf muscles (sitting or standing); (e) trunk rotation (lying or sitting); (f) extension of thoracic spine/shoulder elevation (supine).

Maintaining mobility

Danger times

The person must understand that any period of immobility is potentially dangerous and that special care is required at such a time (figure 3.2). The effect on tone or posture of prolonged rest or confinement to bed, or the reduced experience of movement alone, may just tip the balance when independence is already borderline. Many people lose some functional skill unnecessarily at these times because they have not been told of the hazards associated with reduced activity. Routine stretching must continue and it is important to practise independent balance in sitting and to stand and walk every day.

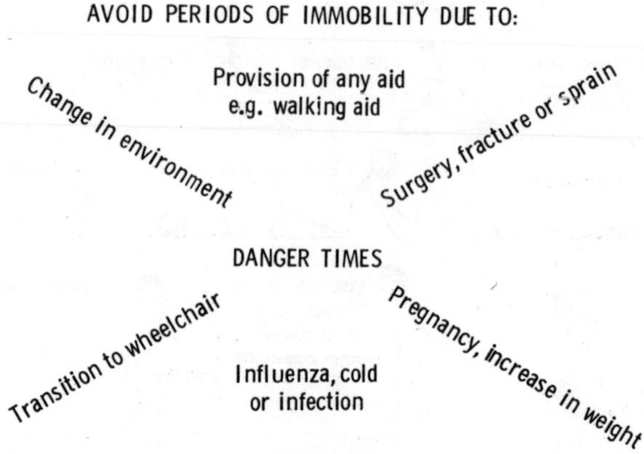

Figure 3.2

At any of these danger times the resulting reduced experience of movement in the presence of abnormal tone or ataxia will result in deprivation of normal movement. This often means that the movement may be forgotten and the ability lost completely. It becomes obvious that extra attention is needed to ensure that an adequate experience of everyday movement is maintained. This will need to be explained carefully to the person himself and to relatives so that such vicious circles are avoided (figure 3.3).

A refresher course of intensive therapy may need to be suitably timed to regain any function liable to be lost during this period.

Abnormal movement patterns

When movement is difficult or reduced, fixed or abnormal patterns of movement or reflex attitudes are often used. Because such solutions are short term and actually lead to a further loss of function, early observation and correction of any abnormal movement patterns will greatly influence both prolongation of independence and the course of future man-

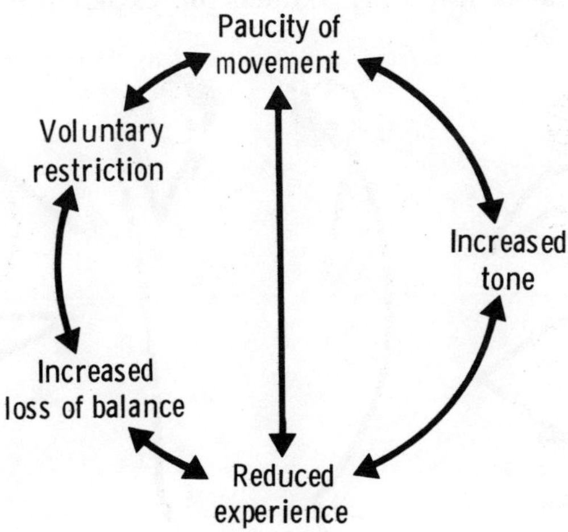

Figure 3.3

agement. Without extra emphasis to stimulate the normal postural and balance mechanisms in all positions and at different speeds in order to keep a good background for the functional use of limbs, other activities in other positions will also be adversely affected.

Examples of this group of reflex attitudes include the following:

(a) Voluntary restriction of head movement, and loss of trunk rotation when walking, will affect the balance mechanisms in sitting, and consequently dressing and feeding skills. It may also mean that turning over in bed could become more laboured.

(b) Continued use of a total extension synergy in the lower limb when walking will contribute both to loss of control of isolated movement and to reduced balance reactions in the leg. This could also hasten the loss of ability to walk at all. If uncorrected, such a walking pattern could eventually prevent transferring in safety and even predispose to contracture in the hip flexors and calf muscles.

Use of typical tonic reflex attitudes (figure 3.4), if not corrected, have somewhat detrimental consequences. Such postures may be adopted either for stabilisation or for movement. Fixed attitudes not only reduce the experience of normal

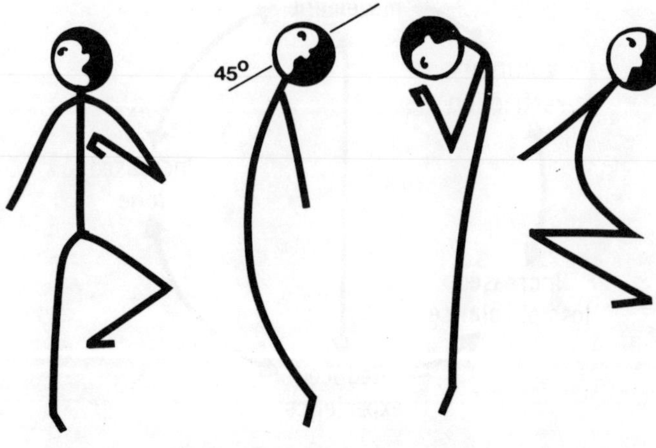

Figure 3.4 Patient in bed showing abnormal postures.

movement and posture when performing functional activities; in time they will also alter the distribution of tone throughout the body and may actually prevent the performance of the movement they were recruited to assist. In addition, they may initiate a vicious circle of complications.

Example of this group of reflex attitudes include

(a) Leaning heavily on a stick, prolonged stabilising with one hand, and controlling a motorised wheel-chair in an asymmetrical tonic neck reflex (ATNR) attitude all tend to increase tone in a typical pattern and if continued would cause loss of function and contractures.

(b) Using a head posture in which a tonic labyrinthine attitude could be influential when standing or walking may eventually make it impossible to bring one foot in front of the other because of the increased extension produced.

(c) A similar effect can be demonstrated if a symmetrical tonic neck reflex (STNR) attitude is used when transferring or when walking with a frame, and is likely to lead to a contracture of the calf muscles.

(d) Propelling a wheel-chair incorrectly by pushing the head into extension could in time contribute to uncontrollable flexion in the lower extremities.

Vicious circles

The many vicious circles which commonly occur will demonstrate the fine balance between easy management and multiple problems (figure 3.5). Unless prompt action is taken at the first sign of trouble, one circle can lead to another in any sequence and with surprising speed.

Examples of the vicious circles which may occur are given below:

(a) Faulty bowel management will increase tone generally, which could reduce function or prevent the ability to walk. This leads to contractures, further increase of tone and sores.

(b) Lying in an unsuitable position in bed increases tone and results in poor function, which leads to sores and contractures.

(c) Sitting with the forefoot in a bad position on the foot-

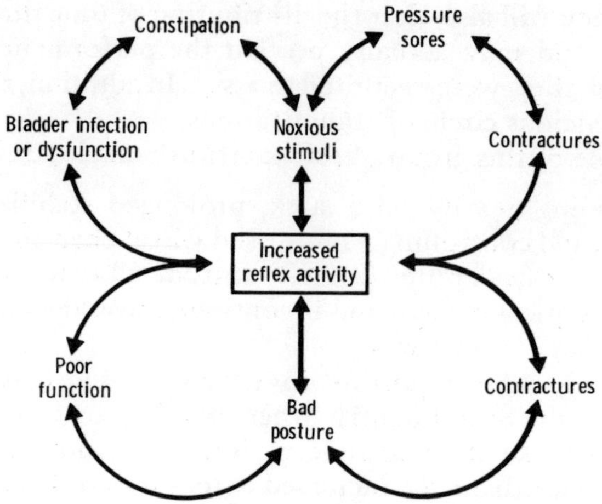

Figure 3.5 Vicious circles.

plate of a wheel-chair allows the toe flexors to shorten. Any tight structure will cause increased tone which could lead to pressure sores and prevention of standing and walking.

Provision of aids

Great care must always be taken over the decision to give any aid to a disabled person, and such decisions are usually more satisfactory when made by several members of the team and the family concerned, so that the possible detrimental effects as well as the advantages may be fully considered. Where possible the aid should be given during a refresher course of therapy to enable adequate instruction and evaluation to be carried out. In no area is this more important than in the provision of an aid for walking. In every case, suitable activities will have to be introduced in order to counteract the inevitable detrimental effects (figure 3.6). As these are not always immediately apparent, arrangements should be made for a further follow-up.

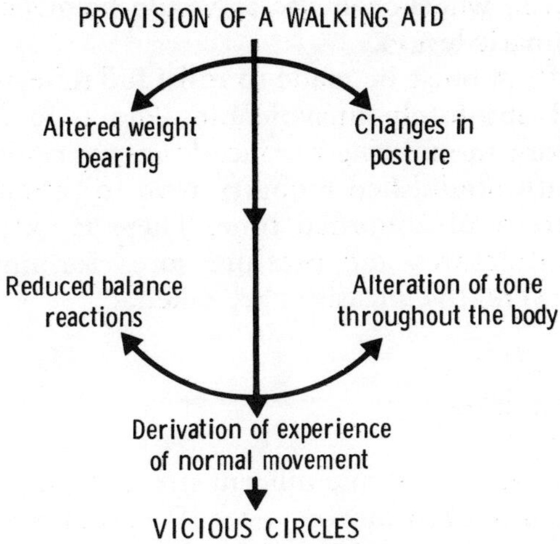

Figure 3.6 Detrimental effects of the provision of a walking aid.

Use of an aid will reduce the inhibitory effect on spasticity of weight bearing through the limbs. Even though gait has been carefully taught, the change in posture can be a shift sideways of the trunk with a stick or forward flexion of the trunk with crutches or a frame. Any walking aid will always adversely affect the balance mechanisms because it reduces the demand for normal head and trunk reactions and will alter the pattern of tone with obvious result to movement. Without the addition of activities which correct and compensate for these detrimental effects, the typical vicious circles will result.

Wheel-chair use

The prescription of a wheel-chair is a most important decision which should involve the whole team, the user and the relatives. It is such a critical period in management and many vicious circles are directly related to insufficient supervision at this time. It is just as important for a person with multiple sclerosis to receive the detailed instruction and meticulous preparation in wheel-chair use as would be given to a person with a traumatic lesion.

Every effort must be made to resist full time use of a wheelchair until absolutely unavoidable. The time of transition requires close monitoring because longer periods in a sitting position with diminished mobility tend to produce a change in the pattern of abnormal tone. There is extra danger of flexion contractures and pressure sores forming unless additional preventative measures are taken.

Recommendations

(a) It is vital to continue diligent stretching of all the muscle groups which tend to shorten, even if assistance is required.

(b) Extra work for stimulation of balance and posture will be required and encouragement to sit in other chairs is helpful, for example at mealtimes.

(c) Continued use of a standing transfer is important and enables an extra stretch to be added each time it is performed, thus helping to maintain full range in the legs.

(d) It is of the utmost importance that the wheel-chair user continues to walk every day. However, for this to be effective it must be in a reasonable manner to ensure adequate weight bearing and adequate stretching of muscle groups. If extra support is required to facilitate this, in the way of gaiters, bracing, parallel bars, etc., these should be readily available so that the routine of daily weight bearing is not interrupted.

(e) Positioning becomes even more important as activity decreases and it is vital that all bad positions should be avoided. Any consistent asymmetry in the trunk or limbs will be the start of a vicious circle of complications; for example, vigilant attention in the correction of sitting posture can often avert problems of head control or balance which may affect speech and feeding. A seemingly minor asymmetry can lead to the most gross difficulty if not corrected.

(f) If walking is no longer feasible, even as a maintenance procedure, provision must be made for a regular standing programme. Some of the physiological benefits of standing are as follows: to normalise tone; to maintain length of leg muscles; to help kidney drainage; to help counteract osteoporosis; to correct posture and any asymmetry.

If necessary, gaiters, plaster back slabs or long leg bracing may be used to support the knees and keep them extended, and if needed suitable apparatus (for example parallel bars or a standing frame) must be supplied to assist standing at home. It is even more beneficial if it can be an active experience by correction of posture, practising balance or perhaps incorporating some diversional activity while in the standing position. In a hospital or in residential care a tilt table may be helpful, but usually tends to be more passive and does not provide quite such effective weight bearing.

Adjustments in management will need to be considered if any of the usual activities in the maintenance programme become difficult or need a longer time to perform, or when full range is difficult or impossible to obtain. A change in emphasis, or additional activities, may be all that is necessary to prevent contracture. Sometimes intrathecal injections of phenol or all-round inhibitory plasters may be useful to keep range of motion at difficult periods. If contractures do occur, application of serial plasters or surgery may be used to correct the shortening. However, without a change in management to avoid the original cause of the difficulty, the problem usually returns.

Summary

Attention to the general philosophy of physiotherapy may prolong the patient's full participation in life and will make him/her much easier to help when functional activities require assistance.

Early assessment by the rehabilitation team enables an appropriate programme for physical management to be incorporated into the daily life. This will be infinitely more effective than two or three out-patient visits a week to the therapy department for a one hour treatment session.

The emphasis should be on the patient to help him or her to educate the family or relatives as to how best the sufferer can be enabled to maintain an independent existence. There should be similar stress of the need for periodic assessments by the rehabilitation team to review the programme and make any adjustments in management or, if necessary, to arrange a refresher course of intensive therapy.

It is better to be in a position to help the patient on a continuous basis than to be called when the condition deteriorates, or when complications have already occurred.

4 The occupational therapist in the rehabilitation team

June Sutherland

In a hospital setting, the aim of the occupational therapist is to strive with the rehabilitation team to get the maximum performance from the patient and to provide practical assistance in the form of aids to daily living, housing adaptations, and advice to the patient and his or her family in preparation for the patient's return home.

For a community occupational therapist, the aim is to ensure that this function is maintained and to try to prevent hospital admission - after all, it is at home that the handicapped person must live and be enabled to take his or her rightful place.

Often in severe cases, where the family are no longer able to cope, or because of bereavement, the therapist can contribute to a complete assessment for nursing care or for future placement in sheltered accommodation, a young chronic sick unit, or a private home.

Assessment

The assessment carried out by the occupational therapist complements the medical assessment of the patient's neurological status and the physiotherapist's assessment of the patient's motor ability. The particular skill of the occupational therapist is to assess the patient's performance in the activities of daily living (ADL). For example, it must be established whether there are difficulties with any of the following:

(a) *Domestic organisation* – meal preparation, laundering, cleaning, shopping, sewing and mending.

(b) *Personal care* – feeding, washing, lavatory use.

(c) *Mobility* – walking unaided, with aid, with help of one person, chair or bed-bound.

(d) *Work* – type of job. Is this full-time, part-time or sheltered work, employment at home, home tuition, diversional outside home, or diversional inside home?

(e) *Transport* – What type is available?

(f) *Home situation* – Who is at home? Is there help from family or friends? What type of accommodation?

In the context of the rehabilitation team, the assessment of home and work is done jointly with the medical social worker (see chapter 6). The construction of a simple social network diagram, as described by Capildeo *et al.* (1976), may be a useful visual aid (see appendix on page 58).

Leisure

Many patients may be denied leisure opportunities because of their disability and travel difficulties. Advice, in consultation with other members of the rehabilitation team, should be offered as to suitable activities. Two useful information pamphlets are available from the Disabled Living Foundation and cover (a) leisure activities and (b) sports and physical recreation (Croucher, 1981).

Remedial activities

During the early stages of multiple sclerosis little therapy is necessary. Once the diagnosis has been made the occupational therapist will monitor the patient's progress in collaboration with the doctor. As soon as there are any problems as regards practical mobility or activity in daily living, the occupational therapist will become involved.

At this stage some patients benefit from short, sharp, intensive treatment sessions on a daily basis as an out-patient.

Activities are chosen to build up strength, general stamina, co-ordination and, most important of all, the patient's confidence in his or her ability to improve. Care should be taken to select activities that do not increase flexor or extensor tone in the trunk or lower limbs, or exhaust the patient, as over-exertion in certain muscle groups can produce clonus.

Doctors and therapists prefer these intensive treatment sessions to be given to patients who are just recovering from an exacerbation: therapy appears to be most beneficial at such times. These treatments are more easily arranged where there is 'open referral' to a department by general practitioners.

Admission to hospital for further assessment and treatment in the rehabilitation department may be necessary if the condition of the patient deteriorates or if members of the family are finding it difficult to cope at home. Attendance at a rehabilitation centre may be for several weeks, where an intensive all day programme of physiotherapy and occupational therapy can be given.

Aids to daily living

Aids to daily living are often bought as a last resort. Many patients may be reluctant to accept aids since they can be taken as an admission of failure. Careful assessment is therefore vital. It is important to question whether the patient really needs the aid, whether it has been tried out, whether it does the job required, and whether the patient is motivated enough to use it without supervision. Careful assessment is also required as many aids are not needed during a remission period. The following should be considered:

(a) *Mobility aids.* The main aim is to reinforce the correct use of the appropriate walking aid, for example stick, frame, rollator or walking trolley.

(b) *Arm-chairs.* It may be necessary to raise the arm-chair on blocks 4–6 inches (10–15 centimetres) in height, or to provide a spring seat.

(c) *Wheel-chairs and extras.* Less than 10 per cent of patients are likely to require wheel-chairs, and initially the patient may just need a light-weight transit chair to go in the boot of a car, in order to accompany friends or family on an outing. Careful reassessment over the years is necessary. Patients with advanced multiple sclerosis may require a self-propelling or electrically controlled chair. In wheel-chair assessment the rehabilitation team must consider three points: (i) the requirements of the patient and attendant; (ii) the function of the chair and extras available; (iii) the environment.

Posture

Posture is very important and should be carefully explained. Faulty positioning in a wheel-chair can affect trunk and lower limb flexor and extensor tone.

If a patient has increased flexor tone in the lower limbs, the correct positioning of the foot on the footplate is vital. The heel should be firmly on the plate. It helps to increase the depth of the heel loop to obtain this. A useful test is to slip two fingers horizontally between the front of the thigh and the wheel-chair cushion. If these slip in with ease the

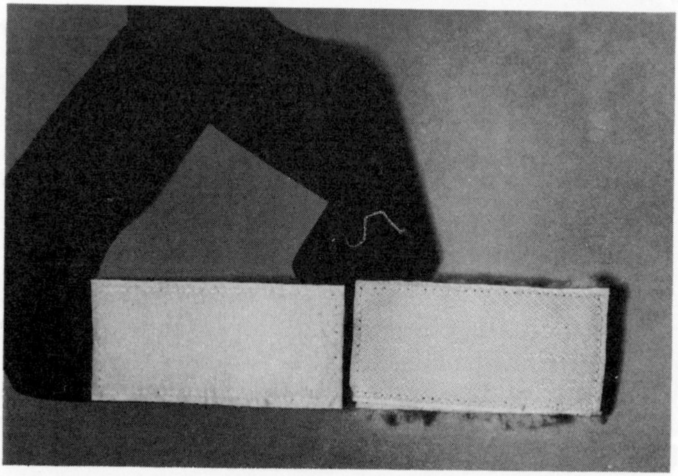

Figure 4.1 The 'Mary Marlborough Lodge' knee strap.

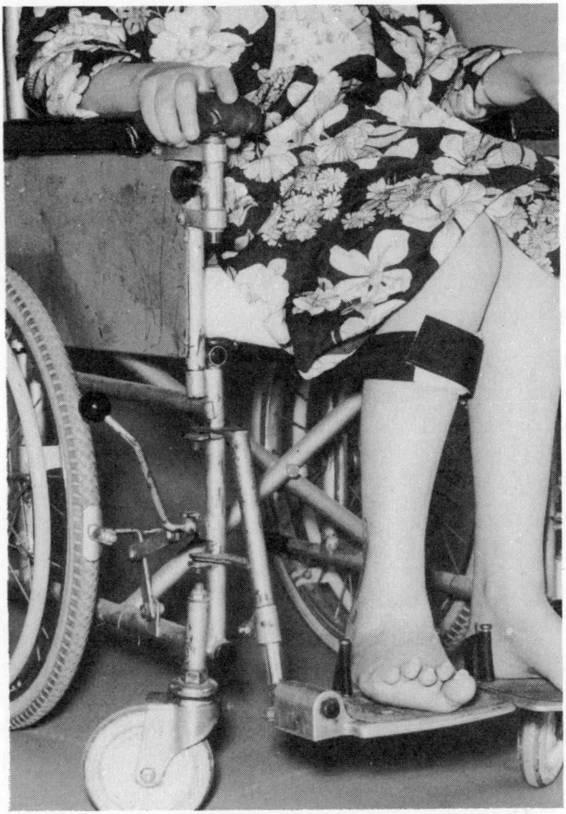

Figure 4.2 The 'Mary Marlborough Lodge' knee strap in position.

footplate is the correct height. The patient should wear his usual shoes – the height of the heel is vital. Often patients are assessed in their best shoes and then wear slippers or no shoes at home. The footplate is then at the wrong height. This will result in an increase of the plantar reflexes, a particular problem in the late stage of the disease.

When clonus is present it may help to insulate the patient from 'jolts' on a rough pavement by providing a cushion. If a patient has increased extensor tone in the spine and lower limbs and, as a result, slips forward out of the chair, the 'Mary Marlborough Lodge' knee straps may help (figures 4.1

and 4.2). These are often successful when body restraining or toe straps have not worked. Also wedge cushions are now being made more frequently for patients.

Comfort

Correct posture should assist comfort. However, it is necessary to provide some form of cushioning. The Department of Health and Social Security (DHSS) provides the following seating cushions:

(a) Foam cushions 2-4 inches (5-10 centimetres) deep covered in vinyl. Plywood bases under the cushion will prevent the seat and back canvas stretching.
(b) Foam cushions 2-4 inches (5-10 centimetres) deep covered in sheepskin which can be removed for washing.
(c) Spenco-gel cushions.
(d) Talley-Ripple Electric motor cushions.

There are also other cushions which can be bought privately. These include: foam, visco-elastic flexible polyester, gel, water, air, alternating air pressure and particle-filled. Some of these cushions may be available in certain cases from the DHSS. The cost varies from £10 to £145.

A careful assessment is needed before purchase. Some firms are prepared to let patients try these on a 'sale or return' basis.

Transfers

Swinging detachable arm rests and swinging leg rests or foot-plates will assist transferring. Extended padded arm rests will help patients doing 90° pivot turns from the wheel-chair to the lavatory or bed. These are not available from the DHSS but have to be individually made. The Rehabilitation Engineering Movement Advisory Panels (REMAP) may help with this: the national organiser is Mr M.J. Marshall, REMAP, Room 37, Thames House North, Millbank, London SW1P 4QG.

A transfer board could be issued if the patient has enough strength in the upper limbs to slide across.

Propulsion

The patient should be encouraged to use a self-propelled chair for as long as possible. If, however, an electrically propelled wheel-chair is necessary, one may have to consider Dudley controls or Malden care proportional control joysticks.

Practice will be needed to build up the patient's confidence. The therapist should not let the patient give up if not successful at first and should provide careful instruction and practice. The therapist should monitor any signs of increased muscle tone in the limb opposite to the hand using the control and make the patient aware of the poor postural position and compensate for it.

Extra wheel-chair features

(a) *Elevating leg rests* are sometimes issued to reduce leg oedema. In general these are not recommended as they do not inhibit increased extensor tone of spine.

(b) *Footplates:* the 8BL footplate can be difficult to swing; the 8L footplate is easier for patients with poor co-ordination.

(c) *Extended footplates* are not advisable as they can increase a patient's extensor tone and make it harder to get the leg back to a 90° position.

(d) *Extended head rests* are sometimes fitted to assist the activities of daily living: for example, when eating, if a head tremor is present. Head rests can stimulate the extensor tone in the spine and are not always suitable.

(e) *Reclining back rests* are contraindicated if there is increased extensor tone.

Hoists

The need for a hoist is apparent during the later stages of multiple sclerosis. There are at least 40 hoists on the British market today. A useful reference is *Hoists and Their Use,* published on behalf of the Disabled Living Foundation (Tarling, 1980). This book gives the dimensions and details of all hoists and guidance on assessment and prescription. Usually the mobile hoists require an attendant to operate them. Care should be taken to teach the method of use carefully and provide supervised practice for the patient and attendant. If the district nurse is involved, then the selection of the appropriate hoist should be considered jointly.

The types available are as follows:

(a) *Mobile:* Arjo UK Pilot; Medihoist; Ambulift (suitable for hospital only); Meccalift (the advantages of this model are that it dismantles when not in use and can be stored under a bed - it will also transfer a patient into a car from a wheelchair). There are three bases: the standard U-base, the Y-shaped base and the static bathroom base. The makes of base are as follows: Zimmer, Steelnurse, Isis, and Autolift (one of the few which can be controlled by the patient).

(b) *Electric:* Winchester-Carters (J. & A.); Master-hoist Carters (J. & A.); Commodore (SML Ltd); Railvalift; Wessex (Wessex Medical Equipment Ltd). Most electric hoist companies will provide a gantry, some up to 12 feet (3½ metres). This usually spans a bed, commode, or space for a wheelchair. It can be used to span a staircase or a long lift model can be provided to transfer a person from one floor to another. All electric hoists except the Railvalift can be supplied with transverse motors to help patients not only move it up and down but also from side to side.

Most hoists require slings. There are seven types available: two-piece sling; hammock with commode hole and divided leg piece; hammock trimmed with sheepskin with commode hole and divided leg piece; divided leg sling; one-piece sling; four-point sling; Lewisham triple sling.

Generally the hammock-type slings offer the most support for multiple sclerosis patients; when patients have to sit on slings for a period of time the sheepskin-lined ones are the least likely to rub.

Driving

Another aid to mobility in less severe cases is the car. In the community many multiple sclerosis patients drive or wish to continue to drive. If in doubt visual accuity should be tested by the hospital and speed of reactions and co-ordination assessed by the British School of Motoring disability training centre. Occupational therapists and doctors in the rehabilitation team may also be involved in the assessment.

Domestic Organisation

The occupational therapist must encourage the patient to be as independent as possible and to incorporate exercises into every day domestic activities. Patients should be told that they will recover with rest if they become tired, hot and exhausted after domestic exertion. The therapist and patient could carry out a time and motion study of kitchen and domestic activities, aiming to conserve energy for those patients who find domestic work tiring.

Tins, pots, pans and china can be moved to accessible shelves. The provision of spike boards, non-slip mats, suction bowl grips, walking trolleys and swivel high-stools for food preparation and ironing may be necessary. Adapted cutlery, plate guards and suction egg-cups may also be useful.

For cleaning, a flexible Flo-mop* will save bending and a long handled dustpan and brush, or a helping hand, will be of assistance when cleaning awkward corners.

In later stages of the disease an automatic door opener and intercom, a Possum environmental control or a safety alarm may be necessary.

Personal Care

Clothing

To try to help overcome some of the symptoms of multiple sclerosis the choice of clothing is important. Easily grasped hooks or zip tags, loose-fitting Raglan sleeves or stretch materials may help. Any adaptations must be made to suit

* Vitoplan Ltd., London, SW18.

individual requirements. Openings should be reinforced with tape, or extra stitching. Double buttons (two buttons sewn together) or buttons on elastic shanks are easier to grasp.

Care should be taken to advise the patient not to sit on wrinkled clothes or hard, bulky seams. For the chair-bound patient a wrap-around skirt and poncho is suitable. In the spinal form of multiple sclerosis, elastic stockings and shoes which give good support are recommended. Elastic stockings will require a dedicated attendant to help get them on.

Lavatory use

The provision of a raised lavatory seat 4–6 inches (10–15 centimetres) high, grab rails fixed to the wall, or a free-standing toilet surround may assist the patient. For someone with poor co-ordination a Toi-lock† lavatory paper dispenser or single sheet packets would be helpful. If access to the lavatory is impossible or difficult, a commode or chemical closet may be placed by the bedside.

In the last resort, for the wheel-chair patient who is unable to transfer to the lavatory independently and has to be left alone all day, there are commode pans and cushions available for the following DHSS wheel-chairs:

(a) *Model 1* non-folding self-propelling wheelchair. When ordering a commode pan state on the order form that a commode cushion is required, otherwise a solid cushion without commode pan aperture may be supplied.

(b) *Epic* electrically propelled indoor chair.

Wheel-chair cushions available are U-shaped paraplegic foam cushions incorporating a sub-seal urinal (male or female).

Two suitable commercially available wheel-chairs are (a) the *Newton*, a folding commode wheel chair, and (b) the *Vessa Cadet*, which is supplied with a commode seat. Commercially available wheel-chair cushions include the Jobst Hydromedica Flotation cushion (a gel cushion) and the Talley Electric Ripple cushion with commode aperture.

† Drainage Castings Ltd., Orpington, Kent.

Incontinence of urine

This has been discussed in chapter 2, but the occupational therapist can offer further advice.

'Nilodor' can be used to mask unpleasant smells. Bladder training can be given with the nursing staff to make sure that the patient empties his or her bladder fully and at regular intervals every 2 hours. Some patients may have to be taught how to empty their bladders using manual expression. Constipation should be avoided.

Assessments can be made for the provision of equipment for personal use such as female urinals, St Peters boat urinals, swan-neck urinals or sub-seal urinals.

Assessments with a district nurse or appliance officer can be made for provision of protective equipment such as urinary appliances and protective pans and absorbent pads.

Many styles of plastic net, nylon and a mixture of fabric and cotton pants and pads are available:

(a) Pull-on pants and pads - for stress incontinence or dribbling, but strong upper limbs and grip plus good balance are required to pull these up.

(b) Open flat pants - for patients with all types of incontinence who have to transfer themselves or be transferred on to the pants and then do them up around them. These are better for patients with contractures or weakness in the lower limbs.

(c) Drop front pull-ons. Again the patient has to be able to pull up these pants but the pads can be easily changed without necessarily having to stand. Nimble fingers are required to change the pads.

(d) Drop front/open flat pants. The patient can transfer or lift himself on to these pants as well as change the pad without having to stand.

(e) Gellulose pads and some one-way fabric pants are available which allow urine to pass through to be absorbed by a pad which is held in position in a plastic pouch outside the garment.

The Bed

The following could be considered:

(a) The provision of a bed board to provide a firm base from which to transfer.

(b) The provision of a monkey pole to assist with transferring.

(c) To give mattress protection the provision of a waterproof sheet, a 3 feet by 6 feet (1 metre by 2 metres) plastic draw sheet across the bed, or a Marathon Dri sheet or sheepskin could be considered.

(d) Anti-pressure electric motor-driven mattresses or beds can be obtained: Talley Ripple mattresses; Medicus air bed; Kellie Simpson Edinburgh mattress. The last-mentioned could be considered where there is danger of pressure sores developing. It is necessary to watch the patient's posture, which is very important because these mattresses can affect the patient's flexor and extensor tone and make his or her problems more pronounced.Transfers can also be additionally difficult from an unstable base.

Bathing

The occupational therapist can also carry out assessments on the need for a bath board, bath seat, non-slip mat, shower attachment, soap on a rope, suction soap holder, tap turners, a shower or bath insert or a bath hoist.

Family support

The family, if motivated, caring and available to help, can provide invaluable support. So often it is the patient who gets all the 'therapy' while the husband, wife or attendant, who is coping valiantly at home as a nurse, physiotherapist, occupational therapist and social worker, feels isolated.

The occupational therapist must always include the 'carer' in all decisions and discussions about treatment and equipment. Attendance during treatment sessions is encouraged and information is given about correct positioning and the danger signs of increased flexor or extensor tone in trunk and lower limbs and how to control clonus.

The carer is also advised to encourage the patient in the correct us of the aids supplied and to know where to return them when no longer needed.

Carers are also encouraged to make full use of facilities and services provided by local voluntary societies such as the Multiple Sclerosis Society, ARMS, and the British Red Cross. Help may also be sought from the local Crossroads Care and Attendant Scheme which is designed to give help to attendants on 24 hour duty, the Disabled Living Foundation and local aids centres. Information is also available on Prestel.

Summary

In the treatment of the multiple sclerosis patient the occupational therapist has an important role in the rehabilitation team. The therapist not only works with the patient but with the family. Correct assessment, the initiation of the appropriate treatment, joint treatment programmes with the physiotherapist, home assessment and the planning of aftercare all require a high level of interaction with other members of the team. The therapist must be aware of the vast array of aids that are now available to help patients and their families and must keep up to date with further technological advances.

References

Capildeo, R., Court, C. and Rose, F. C. (1976). Social network diagram, *Br. med. J. i,* 143-4.

Tarling, C. (1980). *Hoists and Their Use,* Heinemann Medical Books, London.

Croucher, N. (1981). *Outdoor Pursuits for Disabled People,* Disabled Living Foundation, London.

The Royal Association for Disability and Rehabilitation (RADAR) (1980). *Sports and Leisure Access Guide for the Disabled Spectator,* RADAR, London.

Appendix: Social Network Diagram

The patient's home is represented by a box, and is described in terms of a two-storey terraced house, or a fifth floor flat in a tower block: see the example in figure 4.3.

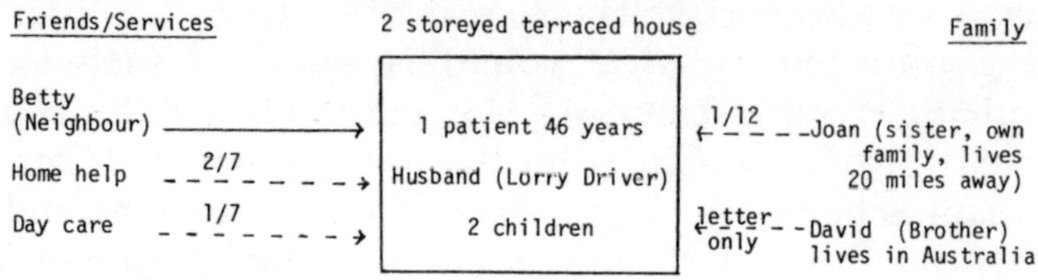

Figure 4.3 Example of a social network diagram (after Capildeo *et al.*, 1976).

In the box, the patient and his or her family are indicated. On the *right* side of the page, immediate family relatives are indicated. On the *left* side of the box, friends and social services are indicated. Daily visits, with directional arrows, are indicated by solid lines. Visits of a frequency less than daily are indicated by broken lines with the frequency indicated above the line in algebraic format, for example 2/7 = twice a week, 1/12 = once a month.

5 Speech therapy and multiple sclerosis

Alison Perry

Although speech symptoms are invariably mentioned in neurological textbooks describing multiple sclerosis, the descriptions are often inconsistent and lack specific detail. The symptoms of this disorder are so varied that they encompass practically the whole field of neurology. Characteristically, in about two-thirds of patients the symptoms come and go spontaneously (exacerbation and remission). In the remaining third, the course is progressive. The possible causes and presentations of multiple sclerosis have been covered earlier, and so will not be dwelt upon: but the classic triad of signs first described by Charcot in 1877 (nystagmus, intention tremor and dysarthria) was first delineated as disseminated sclerosis, today called multiple sclerosis.

The nature of speech problems

In multiple sclerosis, Charcot described the speech as 'slow and drawling', sometimes almost unintelligible, as if the tongue had become 'too thick'. He described the words spoken 'as if measured or "scanned" . . . with a pause after every syllable and the syllables pronounced slowly and hesitantly'. He added that the 'scanning speech . . . may potently contribute to settle the diagnosis, principally in those cases, which are indeed exceptional, where tremor of the hand and upper extremities is absent' (Charcot, 1877, pages 192–3).

Some current neurology textbooks continue to reflect the view that scanning speech is 'typical' or 'characteristic' of multiple sclerosis. However, in a study of 168 patients with multiple sclerosis, Darley *et al.* (1972) concluded that less than half the patients presented with significant speech problems. The most commonly observed deviations were defective articulation, poor pitch control, hypernasality, inappropriate pitch levels and breathiness. Scanning speech was *not* a prominent characteristic of the type of dysarthria which they observed in multiple sclerosis patients.

Multiple sclerosis is often considered to be the only progressive neurological disease which 'progresses slowly enough to warrant a programme of speech rehabilitation' (West and Arisberry, 1968).

Most patients with multiple sclerosis have certain deviant speech characteristics previously described, notably impaired loudness control, harsh voice quality, defective articulation, bizarre emphasis and impaired pitch control.

Speech therapy is geared towards making maximum use of remaining potential and teaching compensatory mechanisms for the impairments. What was previously unconscious in speech now has to be brought under purposeful control. The patient has to be taught to monitor his or her performance continuously, working to see that the standard of speech is as good as possible.

Therapy

Often, listening to tape recordings of his or her speech performance helps to correct deviant production. The earlier this process begins the better. Speech impairment may be controlled by early therapy. The patient is taught to slow down, maintain meaningful stress patterns, and cultivate compensatory movements in articulation of 'difficult' sounds. A realistic treatment programme is necessary, with constant reassurance to the patient that the efforts are worthwhile. It is the role of the therapist to act as a support for expression of feelings of anxiety and depression, as well as offering a practical, structured therapy programme.

Always in therapy with multiple sclerosis patients one aims to keep the patient's speech functioning for as long as possible. However, in recognising that the disorder is progressive, values change and the emphasis is moved from 'speech production' towards 'communication'. This often means issuing a communication aid which will enable the patient to communicate, at however basic a level, for as long as possible.

Methods of assessment

The assessment of dysarthria is now at a more scientific level than ever before. There are various ways in which speech production may be described:

By informal observation

This is a standard part of a neurological examination. A stock expression is often 'slurred speech' - a phrase which apparently overlooks the fact that articulation may be impaired in diverse ways that are of diagnostic significance. Therefore, more standardised measures are needed.

Measurement of simple speech performance

A step further towards objectivity may be to rate a patient's performance on several tasks: for example, asking them to read a set passage aloud and then calculating the oral reading rate; asking a patient to prolong a vowel sound and measuring the duration of maximum phonation; asking the patient to repeat syllables rapidly and measuring the rate of production, etc.

Rating degree of impairment of several speech dimensions

This involves tape-recording patients undertaking set tasks and then listening to brief samples of contextual speech and rating on a scale the degree of impairment in each of several speech and voice aspects, namely pitch, loudness, prosody, etc. This was used in the Mayo Clinic study (Darley *et al.*, 1975).

Objective analysis by instrumentation

One may measure loudness and pitch of voice scientifically using instruments, such as a sound level meter and laryngograph. Palatography allows study of the contact of tongue with the palate and alveolar ridge during speech; intraoral breath pressure may be measured using an oral manometer, together with nasal and oral airflow measurements in speech.

Frenchay dysarthria assessment

Although objective analysis is desirable, one often has a problem in acquiring the machinery to undertake such sophisticated measurement and so a repeatable, easily administered test is essential in order that the same patient's performance may be reliably assessed and re-assessed. One such published is the Frenchay dysarthria assessment (Enderby, 1981).

This consists of subtests of performance on each speech aspect, namely respiration, reflex actions, etc. The patient is asked to undertake set tasks, being tried and assessed on each. A profile is then obtained (figure 5.1) of the performance. It

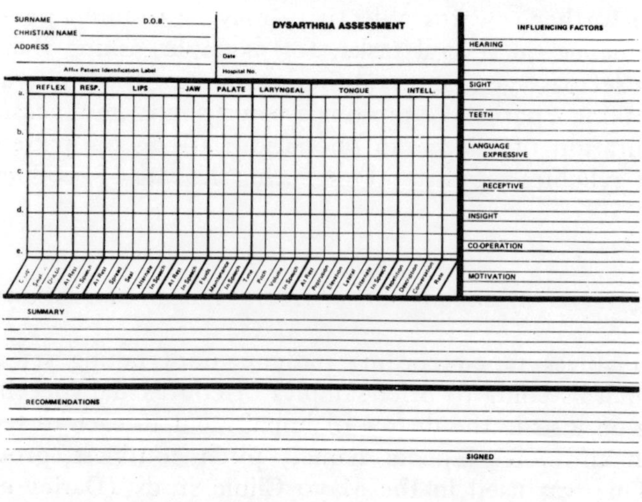

Figure 5.1 Frenchay dysarthria assessment table.

may immediately be seen which aspect of speech production needs remediation – in other words, that which is most detracting from 'normal' communication. Hence, structured testing is vital.

Communication aids

There are various *communication aids* commercially available: four which have been tried and found useful are illustrated in figures 5.2–5.5.

It is impossible simply to issue an aid to a patient. Each patient will need assessment, followed by close instruction to the use of the aid. Whenever possible a choice should be offered of suitable communication aids for patients to be able to decide which is most appropriate for them. Very often patients do not like using a communicator, feeling that this is an 'ad-

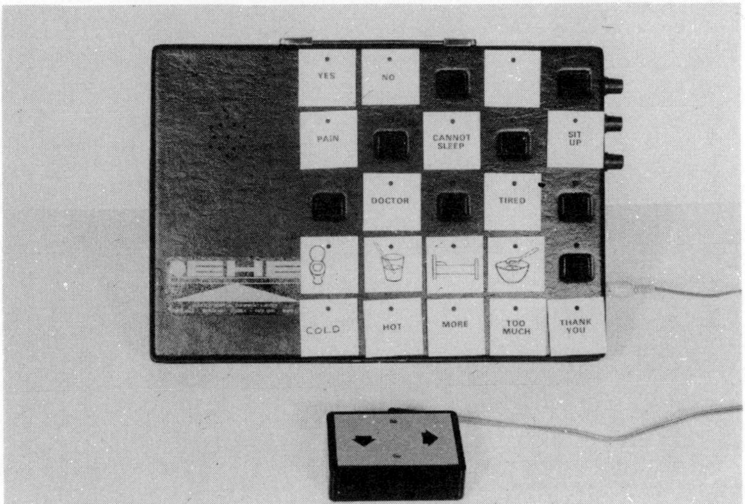

Figure 5.2 An Edu-comm. This consists of a light display board on which basic words are placed. The light can be moved horizontally or vertically across 25 positions by gross hand controls until the desired word is reached. It is suitable for expressing basic needs and wants, and can be operated by mouth with a pneumatic attachment.

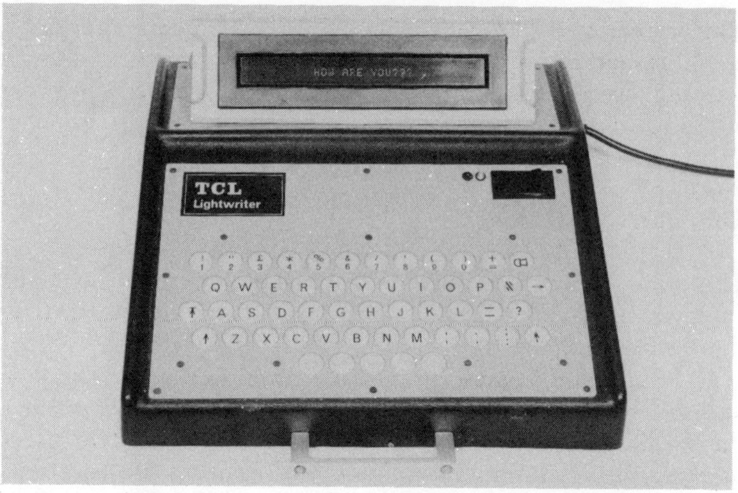

Figure 5.3 A lightwriter. This is similar to a typewriter, but the keys light up on a small screen which can be directed towards the person with whom one wishes to communicate. It operates electrically and the keys are laid out in typewriter fashion, needing finger control.

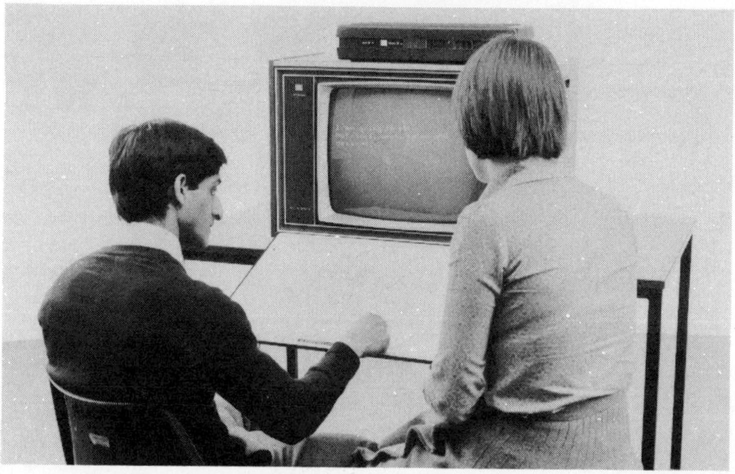

Figure 5.4 The Splink. This consists of a large wordboard (42 mm x 66 mm = 16½ in x 26¼ in) and a microprocessor which is linked to a television set by an infrared process. The board comprises 950 basic words and letters in alphabetical order, together with phrases and numbers. The patient presses a key (2 mm x 1 mm = $\frac{11}{16}''$ x $\frac{5}{16}''$) for the required word, which is then emitted on the television screen. It is not portable because it needs a television set to function; it also demands good scanning ability and manual dexterity.

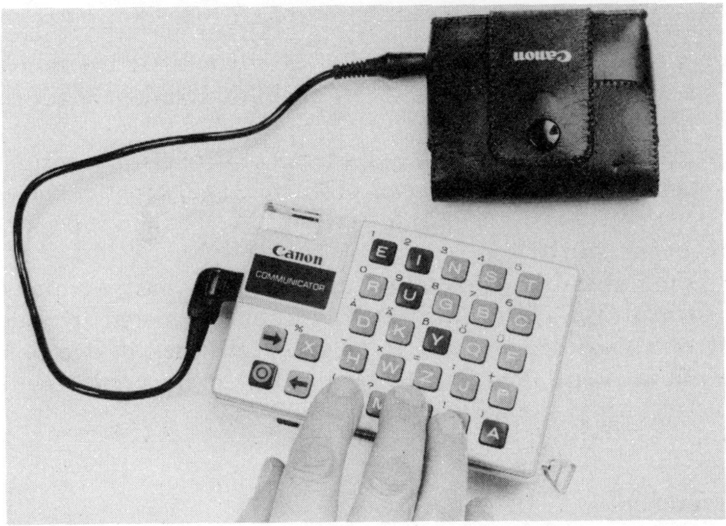

Figure 5.5 The Canon Communicator. This is a portable aid, the size of a pocket calculator, which has letters and a tickertape system. The patient spells out his needs letter by letter, and these are then printed out on the tape. The tape can be torn off and handed to the 'listener' to read. Good visual ability and finger movement are again necessary. If the patient has difficulty with finger co-ordination it is possible to add an overlay to make contact with the letter keys more precise.

mission of defeat'. Provided that realistic but supportive help is given, this attitude may be overcome.

With the future explosion in microprocessors and voice synthesisers perhaps soon the speech aid market will be uplifted by a choice of 'talkers' for patients.

Already '*Handivoice*' is available in the United States of America – this is a voice synthesiser which actually 'speaks' for patients when switches are pressed. However, the Mid-West American accent used does not seem to appeal to patients in Britain so we wait to see what the future may bring.

Summary

Multiple sclerosis, although progressive, is one of the few degenerative neurological conditions which progresses slowly enough to make a programme of speech rehabilitation viable.

The stage at which patients are referred is vital - there is greater potential for conservation of communicative abilities if the patient is referred and treatment undertaken as soon as an initial diagnosis of dysarthria is made.

Early detection, formal assessment and realistic treatment is essential to control speech problems, as the patient needs to concentrate to self-monitor his/her speech, and the sooner this begins the better.

Communication aids have an important part to play in treatment but each aid must be carefully selected to match the needs of each patient. In this way, channels of communication are kept open for as long as possible, thus reducing the frustrations of the patient concerned!

References

Charcot, J. M. (1877). *Lectures on the Diseases of the Nervous System*, Vol. 1, New Sydenham Society, London.

Darley, F. L., Brown, J. R. and Goldstein, N. P. (1972). Dysarthria in multiple sclerosis. *J. Speech Hear. Res.* 15, 229-45.

Darley, F. L., Aronson, A. E. and Brown, J. R. (1975). *Motor Speech Disorders*, Saunders, Toronto, pages 235-48.

Enderby, P. (1981). The Frenchay dysarthria assessment. *Br. J. Dis. Commun.* 15, No. 3, 165-75.

West, R. W. and Arisberry, M. (1968). *The Rehabilitation of Speech*, 4th Edn, Harper & Row, New York.

6 The medical social worker in the rehabilitation team

Christine Randall

The medical social worker is called upon when social breakdown occurs in association with a patient's physical illness. Two contrasting perspectives are involved. First, as a public official of the Social Services Department, and secondly, as a personal witness and confidant to the patient.

Defining the role of the medical social worker

As public officials medical social workers can be considered as representatives of the public response to an individual's illness and disability. They are expected to help the person and his or her family in a time of medical and social crisis by virtue of the fact that they have been trained to know what benefits and resources are available and how they can best be used to assist the person and his or her family in all matters relating to the illness.

This assistance may simply be in the giving or obtaining of information and/or advice. In other situations, benefits and resources are provided according to law but social workers may have to take part in committee in order to decide how these should be fairly distributed. Details of available resources and benefits are included in the appendices on pages 73-83.

The other role of the medical social worker, that of confidant to the patient and his or her family, is considered below.

The patient–medical social worker relationship

Within the context of the rehabilitation team, the medical social worker may gain particular insight into the patient's – and the family's – response to multiple sclerosis. The effects of the disease upon the organs of perception such as the skin and the eyes, as well as more general effects upon body orientation, undermine the individual's confidence, introducing self doubt. This occurs in all cases of multiple sclerosis and results in profound anxiety which permeates all future aspects of life.

The medical social worker in the rehabilitation team

This response to illness is often poorly emphasised in clinical textbooks which deal with the management of multiple sclerosis in a factual way. For example, in Brain's *Diseases of the Nervous System*, under the heading 'Mental Symptoms' in multiple sclerosis, we find the following:

> 'Some reduction in the intellectual efficiency of the patient is not uncommon but emotional changes are more frequent. The characteristic sense of mental and physical well-being – euphoria – is well known. On the other hand, depression and irritability are sometimes conspicuous. Some loss of control over emotional movements, leading to involuntary laughter and tears, is common, especially in the later stages of the illness. Delusional states and a terminal dementia are sometimes met with' (Brain, 1962, page 453).

While this passage gives a synopsis of the observable behaviour, the observations are cold and depersonalised. They really give us little understanding of the 'shock' and personal tragedy experienced by the individual sufferer.

If we approach sufferers in this distanced way we diminish the effectiveness of our other skills in the provision of resources or rehabilitative therapies. It is an important part of the medical social worker's role to allow emotional response to surface. The aim is to give the recuperating patients primary support in terms of their identity, family role and plans for the future. Patients may be referred at the time of a relapse, when the diagnosis can be medically confirmed. Although the patients may have suspected the possibility of this diagnosis for some considerable time, they are 'shocked'. I have been impressed by the degree of emotional chaos displayed at times like this, when the severity of the shock has sometimes produced florrid psychiatric symptoms. Once the concept of 'shock' is accepted, however, the response to illness in psychological terms can be seen as a dynamic process which does not warrant the use of static labels. To illustrate this point two case histories will be described.

Case 1

The patient was a tall, attractive 40 year-old man referred shortly after his admission to hospital.

> 'Four years before referral the patient was married with two children aged 9 and 12 years. He was employed in an artistic occupation where his colleagues described him as "talented and creative". When referred he was unemployed, in heavy debt and living in a hostel for alcoholics. During the intervening four years, whilst he was gradually developing symptoms, he had been a picture of ceaseless activity. For example, his attempts to make a living had taken him around the world on innumerable business ventures, each of which failed and compounded the difficulties of the next venture. His denial of the reality of the effects caused by his physical symptoms led to his subsequent denial of the fact that he was dependent upon his immediate family. The result was that his marriage failed in an atmosphere of hostile bitterness. On admission he was severely ataxic and suffered from double vision. He believed himself to be suffering from secondary brain tumours from which his father had died three years previously. It was the hostel warden who had pressed the general practitioner to see him, because he

was falling about the house when the warden knew that he was not drunk.'

Initially I found the patient to be nihilistically depressed but upon being told his diagnosis he became quite euphoric. For several days he lunged about the ward telling everyone how happy he was that he did not have cancer and made grandiose plans for his future. Earlier referral and more sympathetic follow-up might have prevented this patient's tragic social decline.

Case 2

The patient was a shy man of 46 years, who, when first seen, was severely depressed with bouts of crying and deep despair. He said, 'I have not lived since I was in my twenties'.

> 'At this time his life had been full of activity and ambition, a special girl friend, a teacher training course, further study, playing music and activities such as rowing and sculling. Now, he held a low paid job as a clerical officer in the Civil Service. Other staff in his department were half his age and sexually and physically active. In contrast he lived in a tower block with his 83 year old mother.'

These two clients gave florrid expression to their feelings of shock. Other patients react less severely, but these feelings are not trivial. They are authentic and full of meaning and affect the individual's response to the illness and subsequent recovery.

As well as the effects of 'shock' at diagnosis and during relapse, there are effects upon the chronic ambulant client who is possibly diagnosed retrospectively and has been aware of the condition for a number of years. At diagnosis, as we have seen, he/she is likely already to be undermined and self-doubting. Although possibly relieved to hear that the condition can be given a medical name, he/she has to go on finding out what this means in every day life and what changes will occur as the disease progresses. How can a patient make a 'once and for all acceptance' of a condition that is notoriously liable to relapse?

Elizabeth Forsythe (1979) describes her experience of the transient neurological symptoms before diagnosis:

> 'Looking back now, with the benefit of hindsight, I can remember that I had a mysteriously weak left leg, which started at the end of my final examinations. I do remember that there were some neurological signs in the leg and it was thought that there might be pressure on a nerve in my back . . . . I had periods of fatigue while doing my early resident jobs, I thought excessively. After the weak leg I never had the same resilience again. At times the fatigue was so extreme that I had to stop working for a while. It was never considered that I could have a physical illness but was probably attributed to "neurasthenia" or possibly in more basic language - lack of guts!'

Secondly, she discusses the social consequences in the following extract:

> 'I had wanted to specialise in children's medicine and during my student days was encouraged in this ambition by those for whom I worked. This attitude changed after I qualified and started to have periods of fatigue. Not only did I lose confidence in my own ability but I lost the support of those senior to me on whose help my future would, to a large extent, depend.'

Lastly, she mentions her feelings about herself:

> 'It became clear that I lacked the necessary capacity for hard work to succeed in a competitive profession. At the time I was bitterly disappointed and very depressed at what seemed to me to be failure through my own lack of will power.'

The significance of these passages lies not only in the

undermining self doubt expressed and the shame because of the failure to achieve, but also in her opening words, 'Looking back now . . . '.

Follow-up - support of the patient

Looking back is a very important part of the recuperative process for the client and part of the medical social worker's role is to help the clients to piece together the basis of their lives: who they are, what they have lost, what they want now and what they need. Written social histories are the by-product of this process. Clients should be encouraged to write their own, as recommended by the late Professor Ritchie Russell of Oxford. What is clear is that in the mind of each client the disease means at times that he/she feels robbed of any chance of personal achievement and happiness. It is not surprising that we see clients who are angry and disappointed, their past ambitions already lost and future plans now shattered.

Case 3

> 'The patient was a quick, mentally alert woman who was married with several small children. She made outwardly ambitious and active plans to master her disability, at times in an angry and demanding way. She was a patient who actively sought out the help of the Social Services Department. If her demands could not be met she would become enraged and would then reject *all* help, later telephoning in tears to confess that she was quite hopeless and useless as a wife and mother. After expelling several home helps she finally accepted one who intuitively accepted her and the meaning of her outbursts.'

For some clients the experience is less defeating. One patient that I knew during her periods of remission was able to revive realistic plans for the future. She found a bungalow in a part of the country which she had always liked and moved there with her disabled husband and several children. She organised the architectural adaptations in which she anticipated her own increasing disability and that of her husband.

These case histories illustrate not only the lives of the

patients with quite advanced multiple sclerosis, but also in the different stages of the disease, which starts long before admission and continues long afterwards. We meet patients at different stages both in the progress of the disease and in their emotional responses to it.

It may be difficult to maintain follow-up of each patient. Full follow-up would enable us to observe the patient's response to his or her illness more accurately and to increase the likelihood that he or she will share with us the meaning that the condition has to him or her, enabling our involvement to be more timely and effective.

These pen pictures, portraying aspects of people's lives, are the social experience of a disease which attacks the nervous system in a particularly debilitating way. Despite recent medical advances, patients require practical and personal help, and, in particular, time to recover from the shock of the diagnostic label. They need time to rebuild their sense of self, their role in the family and their future pattern of daily living.

In summary

The medical social worker's role is to accept the individual's emotional distress and to affirm attempts to find meaning, purpose and hope.

References

Brain, R. (1962). *Brain's Diseases of the Nervous System*, 6th edn, OUP, London, p.453.

Forsythe, E. (1979). *Living with Multiple Sclerosis*, Faber and Faber, London.

Appendix A: Practical help

Social services departments

The social services departments were created by the amalgamation of the old Children's Department, Mental Health

Department, Welfare Department or part of a combined Health and Welfare Department which existed in each of the larger local authorities.

The formation of a social services department is the responsibility of each of the following local government authorities: London Boroughs, Metropolitan Districts and County Councils. The authority to form such departments was established by the Social Services Act 1970.

Each of the previous departments had certain duties and responsibilities stemming from Acts of Parliament and the execution of these became the function of the social services departments. These duties and responsibilities have been added to during the subsequent 10 years by further welfare legislation passed by central government. It is important to note that some of the duties and responsibilities imposed are mandatory whilst others are discretionary. The economic climate of the past 10 years has resulted in some legislation appearing on the Statute Book which has either not been implemented, or only partially put into effect. The following Acts of Parliament are those which involve social services departments and are most relevant to the person with a disability. Other relevant legislation which applies to other departments is listed on page 82.

Relevant legislation

(a) *National Assistance Act 1948 (amended by the Local Government Act 1972).* Section 29 of this Act deals with the promotion of the welfare of handicapped persons by local authorities, that is 'persons who are blind, deaf or dumb, and other persons who are substantially and permanently handicapped by illness, injury or congenital deformity or such other disabilities as may be prescribed by the Minister'. Section 30 deals with the use of certain voluntary organisations as agents in the provision of welfare services. Part III allows the local authority to provide residential accommodation, and to finance such accommodation provided by voluntary and charitable organisations.

(b) *Health Services and Public Health Act 1968.* Section 13 of this Act imposes the duty upon local authorities to provide or arrange 'on such a scale as is adequate for the needs of their areas' home help and laundry facilities for households in need of such help.

(c) *Chronically Sick and Disabled Persons Act 1970.* According to Section 1 of this Act the local authorities must inform themselves of the number and needs of the disabled persons in their area, publish information concerning the services they provide, and ensure that disabled persons in their areas are informed of those services. According to Section 2 the local authorities must provide disabled persons in their areas with the following: wireless sets, television sets, library and recreational facilities, outings and educational facilities. This can be done either by direct provision or by giving financial assistance. The same duty applies to transport, adaptation of property, holidays, meals and telephones.

Note: All local authorities use strict criteria for eligibility for such services and small charges are made. These are normally means tested. Adaptations are costly and strict financial assessment is made of the family concerned. Building work is fully costed by the local authority before it is commenced. Local authorities vary enormously in extent of provision and the charges made.

The rationale for the formation of social services departments was threefold: (a) to improve social services for individuals, families and communities; (b) to match more nearly the needs and resources of communities; (c) to reduce the divisiveness caused by placing people's problems in strict categories, according to different departmental responsibilities.

Children's officers, mental welfare officers and welfare officers working under the previous departments became employees of the social services departments and were called by the generic title of social workers. The responsibility of these workers is to fulfil the department's function by personal contact with individuals, families or community groups.

In 1974 the National Health Service (NHS) was re-organised. A consequence of this was that medical social workers and psychiatric social workers employed by the NHS to work in hospitals and clinics became employees of social services departments and therefore of local government. Some local authorities seconded these social workers back to the hospitals and clinics from where they have continued to function. Other authorities removed all the social workers from the hospitals and clinics, thus enlarging the number of staff in the community offices. They offer a service to the hospital as part of the community and not as a separate entity.

Social workers both in the hospital and the community are employed to provide an information and advice service, to carry out certain duties and responsibilities vested in their employing authority and to offer counselling. Individuals, families or groups may themselves approach a social services department and ask to see a social worker.

If an in-patient or out-patient needs advice on any problem, the social work department at the hospital should be approached. A member of the patient's family can also seek advice from the hospital social worker if the matter relates directly or indirectly to the patient's health or illness.

In the case of a patient who has left hospital without contacting a social worker there, it is advisable to approach the social workers at the local office where the patient lives. The address and telephone number may be found listed in the telephone directory with other local government departments, under the name of the local authority.

Third party referrals may be accepted, that is, from those professionally associated with the patient, or by friends, preferably after obtaining informed consent. In some circumstances this may not be possible, but the service offered is confidential and therefore governed by certain unwritten rules. This personal service is given free of charge but certain services offered by the department, for example, home help, 'meals on wheels', or residential care, may be means tested and assessed.

Department of Health and Social Security

This central government department is responsible for health services and the administration of the National Insurance Scheme.

One becomes a member of this scheme by paying *National Insurance contributions*. If in employment, these contributions are likely to be deducted from pay with a contribution from the employer for each employee. If self-employed, certain independent arrangements may be made with this department. The contributions entitle the payee to insurance cover in terms of National Health services, sickness benefit, industrial injury benefit and pension rights. A small part of each contribution also goes towards supplementary benefit. The former group of benefits are regulated by clear rules of entitlement, and eligibility is decided upon the basis of contributions for a specific year or period of time. It is particularly important to note that sickness benefit is not paid for the first three days of illness and that all claims are likely to be paid from the date claimed, unless extenuating circumstances can be shown.

Unemployment benefit is not payable for a period of six weeks if the job has been relinquished voluntarily, as opposed to the person who is sacked, who gets benefit immediately.

Supplementary benefit was devised to offer financial assistace to those in need, who for some clearly valid reason were not entitled to benefit under the other parts of the scheme, for example, those who have not paid National Insurance contributions, school leavers who had made insufficient contributions to receive entitlement, or those whose contribution entitlement had expired, as can happen with unemployment benefit.

Supplementary benefit may also be paid to augment monies from other benefits if certain recognised items of expenditure cannot be met out of the income received. As with the other benefits, payment is only made from the date of the application. Criteria for entitlement are clearly laid down in legislation implemented in November 1980. The effect of this has been to remove the discretionary element which could be exercised by the social security officer, replacing it with a more prescribed tariff system.

Claims made on the National Insurance Scheme must be made by the claimant. It is advisable to make all claims in writing and illness must be proved by the production of medical certificates. In theory claims may be made in person, by telephone or in writing, but when dealing with a large bureaucracy it is advisable to ensure that matters are put into writing. If valuable documentation has to be produced this should be taken in person and a receipt obtained, or sent by recorded letter. The service is confidential.

It is advisable if visiting the office to arrange an appointment as the number of claimants can result in many hours of waiting. In certain circumstances a home visit by a social security officer can be arranged.

The offices of the department are listed in the telephone directory under Health and Social Security. Not all parts of the service may be in the same building. One building may contain pensions and another supplementary benefit. It is important to check that the office with which you intend to correspond covers the area in which the claimant lives. This is less important when applying for unemployment benefit, which is dealt with in yet another office and is administered by the Department of Employment. Part of the requirement for this claim is that the claimant attends in person and demonstrates that he/she is attempting to find work. These offices are listed in the telephone directory under Employment.

By definition it is impossible to claim both sickness benefit and unemployment benefit at the same time. For someone with a severe disability, however, it is important to find out which is the more appropriate benefit.

Each November the rates of payment for all benefits are reviewed and revised whilst supplementary changes may be made during the year. It is important to check the most up-to-date pamphlets concerning benefits and these are listed with reference numbers on page 82.

Help and advice concerning benefits may be obtained from the social security officers. An appeal may be made where a decision is considered unsatisfactory. Help may be obtained in any controversial matter regarding social security from either the Disablement Income Group, the Citizens Advice Bureau or the local Law Centres. These can be found listed in the telephone directory.

Social workers can also advise and suggest local organisations such as welfare rights groups who may be able to give assistance. Some benefits are taxable whilst others are not, and it is wise to seek advice. The following organisation is a registered charity, which acts as a pressure group to give advice on disability and financial matters: Disablement Income Group, 28 Commercial Street, London E1 (telephone 01 247 2128/6877).

Community Health Service

The National Health Service re-organisation in 1974 resulted in a three-tier administration. The country was divided into regions which were composed of a number of Area Health Authorities. A further re-organisation took effect from April 1982. The Area Health Authorities were abolished and the number of Health Districts slightly reduced and some boundaries altered. These are now known as Health Authorities.

The re-organisation in 1974 resulted in the transfer of certain functions from the local authority health departments to the NHS. The rationale for this was to remove the artificial boundaries existing between NHS hospitals and the personal community health services provided by the local authority, for example chiropody, district nurses and health visitors.

The *chiropody service* may be approached directly, although sometimes medical support may be needed, especially if a domiciliary visit is required.

Health visitors and *district nurses* are frequently attached to a group general practice or to a health centre, but sometimes they cover a geographical area individually. They normally have their own office which is listed in the telephone directory under the Health Authority. Patient referrals are normally made by the hospital or general practitioner. Their services are free and home nursing aids are obtainable through them.

Community Health Councils

Community Health Councils (CHCs) were set up as a result of the 1974 re-organisation of the NHS. There is one for each health authority. Apart from a paid secretary, they are generally composed of volunteers: half are appointed by the local authority (London Boroughs, Metropolitan Districts, County Councils and District Councils), one-third are appointed by voluntary organisations (for example Age Concern, Multiple Sclerosis Society or MIND), and the remainder by the Regional Health Authority.

Their function is to represent the interests of the local community, as the users of the health services, to the managers of the NHS. CHCs must be consulted on NHS planning, and the councils have the right to seek information and to visit hospitals, health centres and clinics. They also publicise the services available from the NHS and from time to time put on a study day to provide information on specific health topics. They will also give advice on procedures for making complaints against the NHS. Although unable to take up an individual case, they are in a position to raise issues.

Appendix B: Other organisations

Citizen's Advice Bureau

This organisation is a registered charity with offices in many towns. Each office has its own hours of opening. It is advisable to check these, and although they will see people without an appointment it is advisable to make one. The offices are staffed by paid employees in large urban areas and by trained volunteers in more rural ones. The information and advice which they give covers many areas including aspects of the welfare state, the law relating to housing and employment, and legal matters arising from separation, divorce, custody and maintenance. They keep lists of solicitors, including those who work under the Legal Aid scheme, and will advise on how legal aid can be obtained. Their services are free and they are listed in the telephone directory. Some areas also have Law Centres which are staffed by people knowledgeable on common legal problems who will arrange appointments with visiting solicitors at the centre - this service is also free.

Multiple Sclerosis Society of Great Britain and Northern Ireland

This is a registered charity. Its objectives are to co-operate with the medical profession in encouraging research into the causes and cure of multiple sclerosis and to promote the mutual help and welfare of people suffering from the disease. They keep a register of local branches, of which there are over 330 throughout the country. The head office is at 286 Munster Road, Fulham, London SW6 (telephone 01 381 4022).

The local branches are responsible for fund-raising in co-operation with the parent organisation, and organise social and recreational activities such as yoga and swimming. They offer a personal welfare service which may include financial help with welfare comforts and holidays. CRACK is the organisation for younger people who suffer with multiple sclerosis, but they remain part of the local branches.

Action for Research into Multiple Sclerosis (ARMS)

This organisation was originally a splinter group from the above association. The entire effort of ARMS is put into research (see chapter 8). It can be contacted through the following address: Research Unit, Central Middlesex Hospital, Acton Lane, London NW10 (telephone 01 961 4911).

The Disabled Living Foundation (DLF)

The DLF gives information and advice on all aspects of disability. It holds displays and gives demonstrations of all aids and gadgets. The address is 346 Kensington High Street, London W14.

Appendix C: Brief guide to the explanatory pamphlets of the DHSS

Illness

NI16/Sept. 1980	Sickness benefit
NI16A/Sept. 1980	Invalidity benefit
NI210/Sept. 1980	Non-contributory invalidity pension (men and single women)
NI214/Nov. 1978	Non-contributory invalidity pension for married women
H11/Nov. 1980	Your hospital fares
NI9/Nov. 1980	Going into hospital? What happens to your social security benefit or pension
NI212/Jan. 1980	Invalid care allowance
NHS4/April 1980	NHS dental treatment (also from post offices)
NHS6/Nov. 1978	Your sight and the NHS (also from post offices)

Handicap or disability

NI205/April 1980	Attendance allowance
NI212/Jan. 1980	Invalid care allowance
NI211/March 1980	Mobility allowance
HB1/Jan. 1981	Help for handicapped people (also from local services departments)
HB2/Sept. 1977	Aids for the disabled
NI219/Dec. 1976	Phasing out the invalid tricycle
NI225/Sept. 1978	Mobility allowance: new option for vehicle scheme beneficiaries
HB4/March 1980	Help with mobility: getting around (HB4 is available only from DHSS, DSB7C, Warbeck Hill, Blackpool, Lancs)

General

FB2/Nov. 1980	Which benefit?
NI196/Nov. 1980	Social security benefit rates

NI208/April 1980	National Insurance contribution rates
NI146/Nov. 1980	Catalogue of social security leaflets
FIS1/Nov. 1980	Family Income Supplement (also from post offices)
SB1/Nov. 1980	Cash help: how to claim supplementary benefit
M11/Nov. 1980	Free if you're on a low income: dental treatment, glasses, milk and vitamins, prescriptions (also from post offices)
SB8/Nov. 1980	What happens now you have claimed supplementary benefit
SB9/Nov. 1980	What happens now you have claimed supplementary benefit (if you're unemployed)
SB7/Nov. 1980	Supplementary benefit: living together as husband and wife
OC2/Nov. 1980	Help with heating costs for people getting supplementary benefit
SB12/Nov. 1980	Supplementary benefit: you can appeal
SB16/Nov. 1980	Supplementary benefit: lump sum payments for special needs

Appendix D: Other legislation relevant to disability

Copies of all Acts and other publications listed in this appendix may be obtained through HMSO.

Education Act 1944, Sections 8, 33, 38, 55 and 56
Education (Miscellaneous Provisions) Act 1953, Section 6
Handicapped Pupils and Special Schools Regulations 1959
Education (Handicapped Children) Act 1970
Disabled Persons (Employment) Act 1944
Disabled Persons (Employment) Act 1958
Employment and Training Act 1973
Land Compensation Act 1973, Section 45

Housing Act 1974, Sections 56, 57-84
Housing Rents and Subsidies Act 1975
Rating (Disabled Persons) Act 1978 Sections 1, 2, 3, Schedule 1, Sections 4, 5, 6
Chronically Sick and Disabled Persons Act 1970
Chronically Sick and Disabled Persons (Amendment) Act

Appendix E: Useful information sources

Bell, L. and Klemz, A. (1981). *Physical Handicap: A Guide for the Staff of Social Services Departments*, Woodhead-Faulkner, London.

Darnbrough, A. and Kinrade, D. (1979). *Directory for the Disabled*, Woodhead-Faulkner, London.

Rock, P. (1981). Compass: *Direction finder for disabled people*, Disablement Income Group Charitable Trust, London.

7 The role of diet in multiple sclerosis

M. A. Crawford and Judith Harding

The suggestion of a link between nutrition and multiple sclerosis arose from epidemiological studies which described a high incidence in countries with relatively high saturated fat intakes: in addition, low levels of essential fatty acids (EFA) were recorded in the blood of multiple sclerosis patients (Swank, 1950: Sinclair, 1956: Allison, 1963; Bernsohn and Stephanides, 1976: Dick, 1976). These findings led to a double-blind trial of linoleic acid supplementation in Belfast and London and later in Newcastle (Millar *et al.*, 1973; Bates *et al.*, 1978) which gave encouraging results. The 'linoleic acid' effect is the reason for the current interest in diet and multiple sclerosis, but it is becoming apparent that a case for nutritional counselling can also be made in the interests of the general health of the patients, and that a broader approach might be of more benefit.

Biochemical background and the needs of the nervous system

Fat, along with protein, forms the membrane surrounding each cell in the body. Fat is especially important in the brain and nervous system, since 60 per cent of the solid matter of the brain and 70 per cent of the myelin sheath is lipid. There are different types of fatty acid and their physical properties depend largely on their chemical structure. If a fatty acid has no double bonds, in other words it is fully saturated with hydrogen, it is called a saturated fatty acid and is usually hard, for example, a tallow candle or the solid fat surrounding meat. Fatty acids with one double bond in the chain are called monounsaturated fatty acids, an example of which is oleic acid, very frequently found in plant oils such as olive oil. Polyunsaturated fatty acids have more than one double bond and are usually liquid at room temperature: an example is corn oil, which contains 60 per cent linoleic acid, a polyunsaturated fatty acid with two double bonds.

Just as there are essential and non-essential amino acids in proteins, so there are essential and non-essential fatty acids in lipids. The body is incapable of making EFAs and they must therefore be provided in the diet. There are two families of EFAs: the *n*-6 family and *n*-3 family. In both families the 'parent' EFAs, linoleic and α-linolenic acids, are altered in the body to produce long chain, highly unsaturated derivatives which are vital in the brain and nervous system.

The conversion from parent EFA to active derivative is slow, with 30 molecules of linoleic acid required to produce one of arachidonic acid and 10 molecules of α-linolenic acid to produce one of docosahexaenoic acid over a period of 24 hours (Hassam and Crawford, 1976).

As well as having a vital function as cell-building units, the long chain fatty acids (Crawford *et al.*, 1976) act as precursors of prostaglandins (Van Dorp *et al.*, 1964: Bergstrom *et al.*, 1964; Moncada *et al.*, 1976). The role of prostaglandins in multiple sclerosis has not been fully investigated, but it is thought that they might be important mediators in many of the changes seen in the disease, particularly in relation to the activation of the immune system and their function in maintaining blood flow.

Both families of EFAs are found in the body, where the *n*-6: *n*-3 ratio is 5:1. In the brain the ratio is 1:1. Animal models have demonstrated the requirement for both families in the brain. EFA deficiency in animals has been shown to retard brain development (Caldwell and Churchill, 1966; Galli *et al.*, 1977; Sinclair and Crawford, 1973), alter synaptic function (Sun *et al.*, 1974) and change the electrical activity of the rods of the retina (Benolken *et al.*, 1973).

The complex involvement of the *n*-6 family of EFAs in the nervous system was demonstrated by studies on rats with experimental allergic encephalomyelitis (EAE) (Clausen and Moller, 1967; Selivonchick and Johnston, 1975; Mertin and

Stackpoole, 1978), and the role of α-linolenic acid in nutritional encephalomalacia (NE) in chicks has highlighted the involvement of the *n*-3 series of EFAs (Dror *et al.*, 1976; Crawford *et al.*, 1979). Both of these diseases involve demyelination, and offer evidence that both the families of EFAs may need to be taken into account when considering nutrition and the nervous system.

Double-blind trials

Double-blind trials on linoleic acid supplementation have been carried out, the first in Belfast and London and the second in Newcastle, in which there was a significant reduction in the severity and length of relapses in the treated groups (Millar *et al.*, 1973; Bates *et al.*, 1978). However, in view of the evidence, the balance of both EFA families may need to be considered; so far the trials have examined the effect of only one family - the linoleic acid family (*n*-6).

In addition, since the long chain derivatives of the EFAs are more biologically active than the parent fatty acids (linoleic or α-linolenic acids), an approach embracing both families and their long chain derivatives might be more successful than is a diet containing linoleic, α-linolenic, arachidonic and docosahexaenoic acids. This suggestion has led to the view that nutrition counselling should be available for patients with multiple sclerosis.

Principles of nutrition counselling in multiple sclerosis

The case for nutritional counselling in multiple sclerosis can be made on two grounds - first in the interest of the general health of the patient, and secondly in the more specific interest of the patient's illness.

We have examined the food intakes of 81 patients using a seven day weighed food record method. Two principles seem to emerge. The *first* finding was that food intake in these patients was usually low, which supports previous work (Crawford *et al.*, 1979). However, average calorie intakes for a group of multiple sclerosis patients can be misleading since we have found that the variations between individuals were large. This reflects the fact that some individuals were relatively fit and leading active lives, while others were badly handicapped and unable to shop for food, cook it, or feed themselves. We found that those patients confined to a wheel-chair ate less in energy terms that those who were working.

Some handicapped patients regularly consumed less than 1000 Calories per day. Although energy expenditure is reduced in these cases, weight loss is not common. How much of this weight loss is due to muscle wasting through lack of exercise and how much is due to a dietary deficit is hard to estimate. This view of a low food intake is supported by analysis of blood cholesterol and triglyceride levels, which are consistently below those of age-matched controls (Crawford *et al.*, 1979).

There is an increased risk of dietary deficiencies of nutrients on low calorie intakes. Of the patients whose diets we have analysed, and who were of varying degrees of disability and health, 27 from a group of 81 patients were found to be eating less than the recommended daily amount of one or more vitamins and minerals (DHSS, 1979). The most common nutrients lacking in the diets were folic acid and iron. Even allowing for the reduced requirements of the B-group of vitamins with a low calorie intake, many patients fell below the recommended daily amount for thiamin, riboflavin and nicotinic acid. Recommendation for the essential fatty acids in the context discussed here were not made in the report.

A *second* point derived from the study was the tendency of handicapped patients to rely on foods that are easily purchased, prepared and eaten. Half the patients who had not received any previous dietary advice were not eating salads, 62 were not eating liver and 31 were not eating fish.

Clearly, the volume of food eaten is small, the choice of foods limited, but the nutritional quality of the diet needs to be correspondingly high if dietary standards are to be maintained or if energy requirements are diminished. Multiple sclerosis patients are particularly at risk to major setbacks due to minor infections, including colds and influenza. In the interests of their general health, nutritional counselling would seem to be justified to give the best possible chance of good health and thus the ability to withstand or fight infection.

Nutrition and multiple sclerosis

If nutrition counselling is to be undertaken, one might ask which qualitative aspects of the diet should be emphasised. In our view it makes sense to emphasise those nutrients that are specifically involved in the central nervous system (see Summary). Linoleic acid-rich foods are recommended as linoleic acid is the only agent demonstrated to have an effect on therapy. This means a liberal use of vegetable seed oils and linoleic acid-rich margarines. This recommendation could include the use of salad dressing made from polyunsaturated vegetable oils. The frequent use of green salads with 'French dressing' has the double advantage of providing both linoleic acid in the oil and α-linolenic acid in the greens.

The basic argument presented here is not only that EFA families might be involved but also that the preformed long chain derivatives are used by the brain and should be considered. The rate of conversion of the parent EFAs to their long chain products is slow, and the derivatives themselves are physiologically more potent. Direct sources of the long chain derivatives of linoleic acid can be found in liver, kidney and lean meat. The long chain derivatives of α-linolenic acid are found in fish and other sea foods. They are also conveniently available in cod-liver oil.

In addition to advice on the nature of foods, we recommend, in this context, that attention be given to accessory nutrients. In particular, trace elements such as zinc, copper and iron are components of the desaturase and cyclo-oxygenase systems responsible for the synthesis of long chain derivatives and prostaglandins. The B vitamins are important for chain elongation reactions and this is an additional reason for the regular use of liver. We would include sources of vitamin E and C as important biological antioxidants and because the role of vitamin E is well established in preventing nutritional encephalomalacia. Vitamin E can be obtained from the use of wheat germ and whole wheat or seed foods. It is interesting that one of the beneficial side effects of eating wheat germ and whole grain cereals and breads, reported by the patients, is the greater ease in passing stools. This result is probably a by-product of the increased oil and fibre content of the diet and is quite important to the patient. Vitamin C is also present in association with α-linolenic acid in green vegetables and salads.

Summary

Multiple sclerosis is labelled as an incurable disease. But it follows a course of severe attack, disability and partial recovery. The remission can be long-standing and even permanent. The fact that such remissions do occur suggests that biology has a mechanism which is effective against the disease. This means that there ought to be a way to capture that technique, to use it, or to encourage its success. Nutrition may prove to be one important factor in the management of this disease.

Epidemiological evidence suggests that dietary fat may be involved in multiple sclerosis. Fat is an important nutrient for the brain and nervous system, and in particular there is a requirement for the long chain derivatives of both the essential fatty acids in brain growth and maintenance. Previous interest in EFA nutrition and multiple sclerosis only involved linoleic acid. The evidence now tells us that the issue is more complex. If minor benefits can be obtained from the use of linoleic acid alone, then a more successful approach might be to use both families, their more active long chain derivatives and accessory nutrients.

References

Allison, R. S. (1963). Some neurological aspects of medical geography. *Proc. R. Soc. Med.* 56, 71-76.

Bates, D., Fawcett, P. R. W., Shaw, D. A. and Weightman, D. (1978). Trail of polyunsaturated fatty acids in non-relapsing multiple sclerosis. *Br. med. J. ii*, 932-3.

Benolken, R. M., Anderson, R. E. and Wheeler, T. G. (1973). Membrane fatty acids associated with the electrical response in visual excitation. *Science, N.Y.* **182**, 1253-4.

Bergstrom, S., Danielsson, H. and Samuelsson, B. (1964). Enzymatic formation of prostaglandin (PG)E2 from arachidonic acid PG and related factors 32. *Biochem. biophys. Acta* **90**, 207-210.

Bernsohn, J. and Stephanides, L. M. (1976). Aetiology of multiple sclerosis. *Nature, Lond.* **215**, 821-3.

Caldwell, D. F. and Churchill, J. A. (1966). Learning impairment in rats administered a lipid free diet during pregnancy. *Psychol. Rep.* **19**, 99-102.

Clausen, J. and Moller, J. (1967). Allergic encephalomyelitis induced by brain antigen after deficiency in polyunsaturated fatty acids during myelination. *Acta neurol. scand.* **43**, 375-88.

Crawford, M. A., Budowski, P. and Hassam, A. G. (1979). Dietary management in multiple sclerosis. *Proc. Nutr. Soc.* **38**, 373-89.

Crawford, M. A., Casperd, N. M. and Sinclair, A. J. (1976). The long chain metabolites of linoleic acid in liver and brain in herbivores and carnivores. *Comp. Biochem. Physiol.* **54B**, 395-401.

Dick, G. (1976). The etiology of multiple sclerosis. *Proc. R. Soc. Med.* **69**, 611-5.

Dror, Y., Budowski, P., Bubis, J. J., Sandbank, U. and Wolman, M. (1976). Chick nutritional encephalopathy induced by diet rich in oxidized oil and deficient in tocopherol. *Progr. Neuropath.* **3**, 343-57.

DHSS (1979). *Recommended Daily Amounts of Food Energy and Nutrients for Groups of People in the United Kingdom*, Report on Health and Social Subjects no. 15, HMSO, London.

Galli, C., Galli, G., Spagnuolo, C., Bosisio, E., Tosi, I., Folco, G. C. and Longiave, D. (1977). In *Function and Biosynthesis of Lipids* (Ed. N. G. Bazan, R. R. Brenner and N. M. Giusto), Plenum Press, London, p561

Hassam, A. G. and Crawford, M. A. (1976). The differential incorporation of labelled linoleic, g. linolenic, dihomo-g-linolenic and arachidonic acids into the developing rat brain. *J. Neurochem.* **27**, 967-8.

Mertin, J. and Stackpoole, A. (1978). Suppression by essential fatty acids of experimental allergic encephalomyelitis is abolished by indomethacin. *Prostaglandins Med.* 1, 283-91.

Millar, J. H. D., Zilkha, K. J., Langman, M. J. S., Wright, H. P., Smith, A. D., Belin, J. and Thompson, R. H. S. (1973). Double-blind trial of linoleate supplementation of the diet of multiple sclerosis. *Br. med. J. i*, 765-8.

Moncada, S., Gzyglewski, R., Bunting, S. and Vane, J. R. (1976). An enzyme isolated from arteries transforms prostaglandin endoperoxides to an unstable substance that inhibits platelet aggregation. *Nature, Lond.* 263, 663-5.

Selivonchick, D. P. and Johnston, P. V. (1975). Fat deficiency in rats during development of the central nervous system and susceptibility to experimental allergic encephalomyelitis. *J. Nutr.* 105, 288-300.

Sinclair, A. J. and Crawford, M. A. (1973). The effect of a low-fat maternal diet in neonatal rats. *Br. J. Nutr.* 29, 127-37.

Sinclair, H. M. (1956). Letter to the editor: deficiency of essential fatty acids and atherosclerosis. *Lancet, i*, 381-3.

Sun, G. Y., Go, J. and Sun, A. Y. (1974). Induction of essential fatty acid deficiency in mouse brain: effects of fat deficient diet upon acyl group composition of myelin and synaptosone-rich fractions during development and maturation. *Lipids* 9, 450-4.

Swank, R. L. (1950). Multiple sclerosis, a correlation of its incidence with dietary fat. *Am. J. med. Sci.* 220, 421-30.

Van Dorp, D. A., Beerthuis, R. K., Nugteren, D. H. and Vonkeman, H. (1964). Enzymatic conversion of all-cis polyunsaturated fatty acids into prostaglandins. *Nature, Lond.* 203, 839-41.

8 The role of voluntary organisations

John Simkins

Voluntary organisations have been very successful in their efforts to help the multiple sclerosis patient and to promote new areas of research.

As many as five million people are involved in voluntary work on a regular basis in the United Kingdom according to a recent estimate. The voluntary movement is therefore one of the greatest potential resources that the country possesses.

What are 'voluntary organisations'? Why do they exist, who joins them, what are their goals, how do they operate, what do they achieve, and how can they help in the process of rehabilitation?

Volunteers become involved for a variety of reasons. Some to promote their own image, but mostly to help others, particularly when the volunteer is intimately involved. The volunteer decides to become involved either to bring about change, or in the case of multiple sclerosis to help those affected and to raise funds for medical research to find the answer and, we hope, a cure.

The influence of social change

The rapid social changes over the last 25 years have put voluntary workers into an entirely different role from that of the past when voluntary 'welfare' work was an individual task. Today there is little chance of the individual being really effective unless he or she is part of a corporate effort – a voluntary organisation. This suggests that there has been a levelling down in individual effectiveness rather than a levelling up.

We have seen our official services become more impersonal. The unprecedented pace of change makes demands unknown to our workers of good deeds in the past and there is the steamroller approach of 'authority' to think about. People ask, 'How can I be heard - I have something I want to say that is important for me and my neighbours?'

In general, if they expect to be heard, to be received attentively in this day and age, then they have to group together. A lot of 'fuss and noise' is often necessary, using the numerical strength of a group in order to get a sympathetic response from those who make important decisions for us. So it is the pressures of living in an apparently supportive society that encourage people to band together to form an action group devoted to a specific medical need, because they feel that this need has not been met. Today, there is yet another potent stimulus, that of the government, which encourages voluntary bodies to become involved in many areas hitherto restricted to professional workers.

Types of voluntary organisation

Most people could name a few well-known bodies: for example, Oxfam, the RSPCA, the Spastics Society, or the British Red Cross Society. Some, with special interest or knowledge, could name smaller groups concerned with, for example, speech-impaired children or Huntington's chorea.

There are over 100 groups described as 'voluntary' working in the general medical field. There are large differences between them in terms of organisation and aim. There is the very real question of how 'voluntary' they really are. Can a very large organisation with a central office, paid officials and perhaps a team of field workers in one capacity or another, be termed 'voluntary'? Is it as correct a description for that kind of organisation as it is for the group of volunteers with no paid help, no central office, and in which the field workers are the volunteers themselves?

Whatever our opinion, it does make a difference - a difference in commitment, a difference in the way in which they approach the job, a difference in how and when they make their services available. We should all be concerned when making donations to a voluntary organisation that the proportion of the money spent purely on administration costs is kept as small as possible and that the highest possible share is used directly in progressing the real work of the organisation.

What do the volunteers achieve?

This varies, of course, from group to group, and it depends on what they set out to achieve. Do they have a long term or a short term aim? Do they expect to be very short lived and to achieve just one small objective, or do they expect to develop a long term plan, with continuous activity? Can they cope with the decisions required when faced with the problem perhaps of having won a battle only to discover they are likely to lose the war? The well organised voluntary group knows well that from time to time it may be necessary to lose a battle in order to be sure of winning the war. Who is the enemy? It should not be Government agencies, the DHSS, Social Services, etc., but, in the case of multiple sclerosis, the disease. However, on an individual level, when a patient requires help, the battle may be to get these agencies to provide the care which by law they should provide. Most volunteers see their work as a battle. Achievement is for them the goal, the stimulus, the motivation, the encouragement. Without it the organisations are in danger of disappearing. An ample diet of encouragement in the form of measurable progress is required.

Therein lies another feature of the voluntary organisation: volunteers stop when the need ceases or when the work goes sour. Without the incentive, they stop.

Activities of voluntary organisations

These can be summarised as follows. They raise money. They build houses, laboratories, even monuments. They buy equipment in the face of lack of financial resources from 'official' channels. They create needed services, and sponsor research.

They can get projects moving through sponsorship and can show short cuts and ways to reduce waste. They remind everyone that people are individuals with individual needs - a concept often overlooked these days.

If we want to have a sound appreciation of voluntary organisations we should understand how they operate. Some use the purely physical approach - jackets off and get to work - whether that be building a new school swimming pool or joining a march or a protest demonstration. Perhaps they visit, shop, clean and cook, or take people out on holiday. They may build, mend and decorate. They provide a service just by being there.

Others see their job as much more one of planning, scheming, consulting and development. They supervise and manage, they create opportunities, they seek positive partnership and they expect to be taken seriously.

How do voluntary groups fund themselves?

This is a vital question in times of recession. The first requirement is that they should be confident of success. Once they begin to doubt their own ability they are lost. Given the necessary confidence, funds can be raised through subscriptions, personal donations, and by a myriad of money-raising activities, from the coffee morning to the major celebrity event with masses of media coverage. Some groups obtain grants from companies and charitable trusts, and from government sources.

But for the truly voluntary people it is a case of making an opportunity to help themselves, to provide what resources are necessary to make happen what they want to happen, to participate in designing and manufacturing their own future.

In Britain in the early 1970s, a great deal of research was done which might have led to a major discovery of use to people with multiple sclerosis. Very little of what was done could be termed 'new' work, and was confined strictly to the regular medical disciplines. The approach to research could be regarded as stereotyped. Worse still, information given to patients about their disease was negligible. Very few people were told what their ailment was. There was little or no advice on what they might do about their condition. The vast majority usually found out when it was too late to make the most of their remaining active life. Generally speaking, doctors' responses to their multiple sclerosis patients were patronising and singularly unhelpful, probably because they knew that there was nothing they could do.

People were encouraged to visit a neurological clinic annually, or possibly every 6 months if their relapses were more frequent. In between, they were left very much to their own devices. The only authorised treatments were, and still are, merely symptomatic. The use of steroids often meant that side effects made the patient worse. Counselling was minimal. There were, until comparatively recently, no counsellors trained specifically to deal with multiple sclerosis sufferers or their families and dependants. Rarely, if ever, was it thought that the families needed help. Unfortunately this situation has not greatly changed.

There was a growing unrest amongst multiple sclerosis patients and their relatives who, through a lack of positive information and the clumsy response of authority to their inquiries, had no way of understanding what was being done for them and to them.

Prompted by a controversial press article, 30 people, unknown to each other until that time, met and decided to form a group, subsequently named ARMS (Action for Research into Multiple Sclerosis). The aims were as follows: (a) to stimulate new research projects; (b) to inform and educate multiple sclerosis patients and their families into a better understanding of the disease and of how it could be more effectively managed; (c) to tell the general public about the disease and to increase awareness of its cost in both human and economic terms; (d) to operate a telephone counselling service for multiple sclerosis sufferers to fill the gap left by the limitations of local counselling availability.

The organisational structure of ARMS defined three fundamental rules: (a) that a committee should be formed comprising entirely people directly involved with multiple sclerosis (patients and relatives); (b) that ARMS should not engage in local welfare work; (c) that ARMS should remain an entirely voluntary, self-help organistion with no paid officials or staff.

Since the setting-up of the organisation seven years ago, ARMS has now raised its commitments to £165 000 annually towards medical research. The individual patients and their families receive a regular magazine and a telephone counselling service is constantly manned.

What do the voluntary organisations offer?

At the worst they can, and sometimes do, offer aggravation: time-consuming demands for action which require consideration and decisions. They can force officials to make decisions when they would rather not - sometimes not a good thing when the decisions made are the wrong ones.

At the best a very different result can be achieved. Voluntary organisations can offer a productive co-operation in rehabilitation. They can offer skills that are in high demand, practical assistance in most stages of the work, and opportunities for expression of genuine concern for improvement.

Conclusion

We have learned much in the last seven years about working together with nothing to bind us but a common purpose. There are no sanctions to impose, and people are free to come and go as their physical capabilities and consciences dictate. Despite their handicaps and often distressing symptoms, members consistently respond to a leadership that insists on a programme of creative progress and on the inestimable value to the patient of constructive self-help.

We have all learned a lot about ourselves and the meaning of voluntary commitment. On the way we have each made many friends. In fact, our speciality is the Friends of ARMS group, a number of branches of which are firmly established around the country. These groups are solely concerned with raising money, at which they are remarkably successful.

There can never be a magic formula for success in running a voluntary organisation. However, for us, certain key factors are clearly indicated as essential: (a) a firm, skilled, and sensitive leadership; (b) a confident but questioning membership suffering from limitless enthusiasm; (c) a busy programme regularly throwing up fresh 'high spots' of excitement and interest; (d) well presented information designed to stretch the majority just enough to provide challenge; (e) a businesslike approach to raising funds in which the group's commitments are high, but are presented in such a way that individual members are motivated to set their own targets.

9 Progress in rehabilitation of multiple sclerosis

C. D. Evans

Although there are many beguiling theories as to the nature of multiple sclerosis, its aetiology is not yet established. We know it to be a disease of temperate zones, but even within these it has a widely varying incidence. At the moment infection, heredity, immunology and diet - with particular reference to fatty acids - have all been suggested as possible causes, but none has been confidently accepted or rejected. Prevention is currently impossible and no specific treatment to combat the underlying disease has been developed. The treatments that do exist - steroids, anti-spasmodics, surgery, electrical stimulation, physiotherapy - are at best palliatives, and their effectiveness is uncertain.

A great deal of research is being done to help unravel the problem. Only when the cause has been established can effective treatment and prevention be developed. For the moment the problem remains, and is likely to stay for the foreseeable future. The difficulties experienced by those who suffer from multiple sclerosis have to be dealt with now within our present knowledge. The best strategies must be worked out to help the patients and their relatives to cope with the disease and its effects.

Medical approach

The *first symptoms* of the condition may be episodes of weakness in a limb, altered sensation, bladder trouble, blurred vision, loss of balance or any of the protean manifestations of this condition. At this stage the patient will probably visit the general practitioner for advice regarding the symptoms. The general practitioner's first problem will be to decide whether there is any significance attached to the presenting symptoms, since in isolation each symptom usually means little.

During the *first consultation* an innocent label will probably be attached to the symptoms and the patient reviewed later. It frequently happens that when the patient comes to see the general practitioner next, the symptoms have gone, so no further action is taken. There is also the problem that within the average practice it is unikely that there will be more than two or three patients who suffer from the condition, so multiple sclerosis may not be considered as a diagnosis. Even when the general practitioner may suspect that multiple sclerosis is the cause of the symptoms, he may also consider that referral to a neurological department at this stage would be inappropriate. He would be aware that establishing a diagnosis would be impossible even with hospital facilities. Since there are no definite treatments to be offered, referral may be irrelevant, although when several episodes, separated in time and space, have occurred, or the symptoms become obtrusive, reference will normally be made to a neurological department.

When *referral to hospital* has been made for the purpose of establishing a diagnosis, a full clinical, radiological and serological examination will be carried out together with other available specific tests (see chapter 1). Even then, it is difficult to make a positive diagnosis on other than clinical grounds, since specialised confirmatory tests are outside the scope of most departments. The resulting uncertainty will be reflected in two significant ways: (a) no diagnosis will be given, although suspicions may be voiced to the general practitioner; (b) the patient may be asked to re-attend the neurological departments at regular intervals.

The motives behind both responses are understandable but the impact on the patient may be disturbing. The uncertainty felt by the hospital communicates itself to the patient and will not be reduced by the necessity for continual review. Such reviews are frequently left to junior staff who change rapidly, and their relative inexperience may serve to increase, rather than decrease, the lack of confidence.

When the *diagnosis is definite*, that is after sufficient episodes have occurred to make a positive clinical diagnosis, the patients or their relatives are told. The delay seems inevitable but to many people it appears that the hospital is uncertain, disinterested or possibly mismanaging the condition. Giving the diagnosis of multiple sclerosis is hard: receiving it harder. Much despair, bitterness and anger is generated when it is done. When multiple sclerosis is diagnosed, positive support is essential. Accommodation, jobs and provision for the family may be in urgent need of examination. Advice on how to use community resources is often patchily available, if at all.

There is no measure of *activity of the disease* other than by watching the progress of the symptoms, so that all treatments are geared to relieving symptoms or, put another way, reducing handicap. Incontinence, spasticity, impaired balance, weakness, loss of sensation, and visual and speech disturbances may all need help, so that a wide range of disciplines may be involved in management.

Approach to therapy

One distressing symptom, spasticity, will illustrate our approach to therapy and subsequent pitfalls. Spasticity reflects increased tone, and the patient may have a wide range of symptoms from mild stiffness of an arm or leg to the most disabling flexed and contracted limbs. These present major problems in daily living. Doctors can try to treat spasticity with drugs such as Lioresal, Dantrolene or Diazepam but are frequently unable to judge their real effectiveness in relieving symptoms. For example these drugs can reduce spasticity, as judged by clinical evaluation, and may well reduce the tone and spasms felt, but the ensuing drowsiness and weakness may render the patient more handicapped.

Surgery may help to reduce contractures, electrical stimulation may be tried, and paramedical professions recruited to help. Establishing the effectiveness of such costly regimes is extremely difficult. The costs can, to some extent, be quantified, but the benefits they produce cannot. In part this dilemma arises from our inability to separate natural remission from response treatment.

Other problems stem from the use of inappropriate assessment of the situation. From the medical profession's point of view, the quality of tone, reflexes and the range of movement are all legitimate indicators of the effectiveness of drugs. From the patient's point of view it is more important that the effect of these regimes is greater independence. Establishing the benefit which accrues from this independence is difficult and very subjective.

The medical professions are more orientated towards the diagnosis of the disease than to the amelioration of handicap. If there were better assessments made of handicap and the effect of different regimes, then some progress could be made in determining which is the most effective.

Assessment

During the course of multiple sclerosis in a patient many assessments may be done. Some of these will be relevant, others not. Before any assessment is undertaken the assessor should have a clear idea of the purpose of each piece of information gained. It is important to separate the detailed and sometimes redundant assessments associated with research from practically based assessments which will assist day to day management. Some assessments are carried out by medical staff, others by the paramedical professions.

All assessments should be *reproducible, repeatable, recordable, retrievable* and *relevant*.

If properly designed an assessment should produce the same result whoever makes it, that is it should have no inter- or intra-observer viability. To be *reproducible* there will need to be a fixed protocol or questionnaire, leaving as little room as possible for individual bias to be incorporated into the final result. Assessments need to be *repeatable* so they can be done at successive periods but without the patient 'learning' the task. If the assessment has been indifferently designed, it is possible to demonstrate a spurious improvement through 'practice'; an example is the learning of the 'correct' answers in a set of tests used for psychological assessment.

It is crucial that any information gathered should be capable of clear *recording* and easy *retrieval*. Most methods available have their advantages and disadvantages. A narrative report is easy to make but subject to bias and difficult to retrieve. Graphic display and tightly scheduled examination procedures reduce bias but may increase time in recording. The use of closed-circuit television may produce an accurate picture of a patient at any given time but is costly, time-consuming and difficult to evaluate. These difficulties indicate an area in urgent need of further research.

Finally, it is important that any assessment should be *relevant* and give an accurate representation of the handicap sustained by the patient, allowing consistent management to emerge from the assessment itself.

Rehabilitation concepts

'Rehabilitation' is an over-used word but an under-used concept. It might be more appropriately used if the different types of rehabilitation could be more clearly defined. It is suggested that there may be three aspects to the process.

The *first* aspect is the attempt to reduce the handicap by giving specific treatments in the hope that this will reduce the spasticity, incontinence or other symptoms.

The *second* aspect is where it is recognised that only a limited amount of progress will be made along those lines and that some attempt must be made by means of aids and appliances to modify the environment so that the handicap is less intrusive.

The *third* aspect is the recognition that in spite of individual treatment and aids the handicap has not been relieved. It is at this stage that the modification of attitudes of the patient, those who care for him and, indeed, society at large is needed so that a greater acceptance of the inevitable can be achieved.

Patterns of disease

There are two basic models of handicapping disease.

The *first* model is illustrated in figure 9.1 and shows the

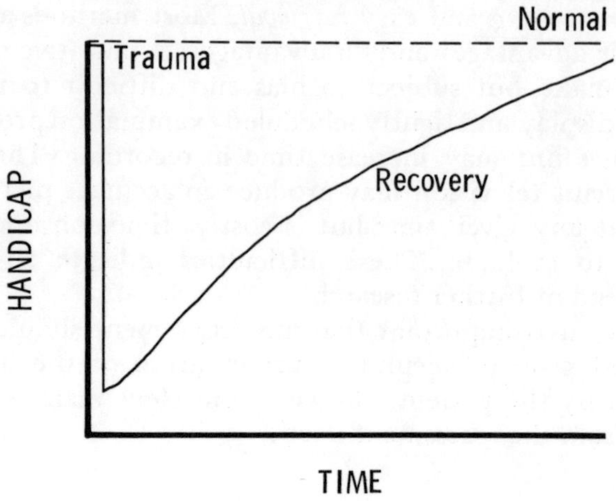

Figure 9.1 An acute illness (such as trauma) with recovery.

case in which a person is involved in some sudden episode such as stroke, trauma or the acute onset of a medical condition. He/she is plunged from being fit and able to a level of complete dependence. From this, depending on the condition and its management, the patient emerges in a gradual curve, the steepness of which implies the rate of recovery. The final height reflects the level of remaining handicap. Fortunately, the vast majority of conditions that are encountered both in general practice and in the hospital allow a complete recovery.

The *second* model includes many conditions, such as multiple sclerosis, which pursue a chronically deteriorating course punctuated by remissions and relapses. This is shown in figure 9.2.

Here the sufferer starts at a level of complete independence and the disease may be present for weeks, months or years before the appearance of symptoms. Further time may elapse before any substantial level of handicap appears. Even when using such models it is not possible to see the effects of intervention clearly. This is another field in which little research has yet been done. Where enough patients with the condition have been followed, however, a pattern of the course of the disease should emerge which may be valid for an individual

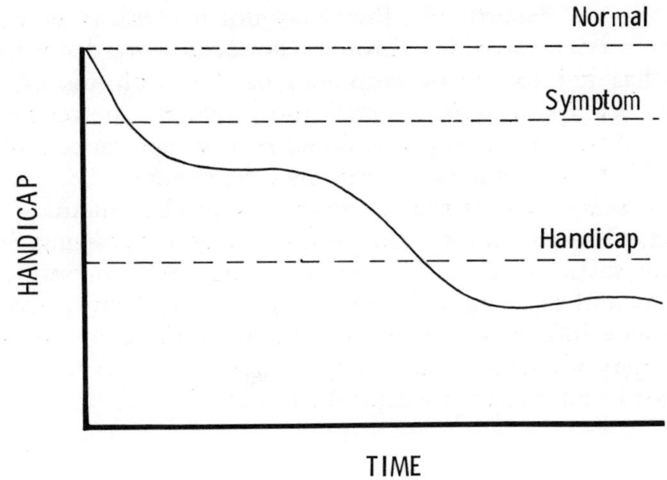

Figure 9.2 A chronic illness (such as multiple sclerosis) with remissions and relapses.

and is likely to be valid for populations. When such baselines have been established, the effect of intervention, be it medical, surgical or therapeutic, might be more readily demonstrated.

Figure 9.2 can also be used to demonstrate the response that the medical profession may have to the patient (see page 102).

The *first stage*, in which there are symptoms but little handicap, corresponds frequently to the initial contacts being made with the general practitioner.

The *second stage* is initiated when symptoms have become specific enough for diagnosis to be established and where a wider range of support and treatment will be offered. The hospital, rehabilitation centre, practitioner, community nurse and social worker may all be involved at this stage. In theory, their job is to make available all relevant services, so they should act as a gateway to greater independence. However, because of the need for economy, even those patients and relatives who know what they want may see the professions as providing a barrier rather than a gateway. Frequently, too, one discipline does not know enough of what another has to offer. If the prime care of the patient is in the hands of a neurological department, they may not necessarily be aware of the services provided through the social work department. This has led to the development of the 'multi-disciplinary team'. At best this works well and provides a better service than before, but inter-professional rivalry, ignorance and the need for economy may mitigate its effectiveness.

The *third stage* is that at which the level of handicap has increased to the point of intruding on day to day living. Some of the difficulties may be from immobility, incontinence, feeding and dressing or from holding down a job and providing economic independence for the family unit. Later the symptoms may progress to the point at which it is difficult for the patient to be cared for within the home.

Approach to community care

Where the care is being maintained in the community it places a long and difficult load upon relatives, friends and other caring staff. It is remarkable in how many cases it is successful. It is essential that those who are involved in the care should be informed of their rights to the allowances and facilities which are legally available. Organisations such as the Multiple Sclerosis Society play a significant role in making sure that its members are aware of their entitlements where general practitioners and hospitals don't give enough information. Some patients are reluctant to join the society because it adds emphasis to the diagnosis which they would prefer to reject. In the same way, many patients will lurch unsteadily round their rooms and houses rather than accept the indignity of a wheel-chair. As some put it, 'I know that once I am in that wheel-chair, I'll never get out'. Their feelings may be right, but it sometimes places an unfair load on those who have to do the caring. Provision of long term care will, ideally, be in the community, with all the support that can be mustered.

Community care sometimes fails and it is a sad fact that those who suffer from multiple sclerosis are one of the largest groups seeking admission into long stay residential care in the United Kingdom. The need for long stay care does not always arise from the increasing handicap of the patient. The health of caring relatives may fail, or they may have to leave the area because of job commitments. The marriage may break up and separation or divorce follow. Some patients prefer to go into care rather than feel a burden to their family. But finding a suitable place in residential care is far from simple.

Residential care

The responsibility for long stay care within the United Kingdom is shared between the social services departments and the National Health Service. The present situation is grim, despite all attempts to improve it. Problems have been caused by the haphazard way that long stay care has developed and by the financial constraints of residential care. The latter depends on who are the sponsors.

Where the social services departments provide residential accommodation, house, contents and most savings have to be given up. Only a relatively small sum of capital can be retained and all taxable income will be taken by the caring unit, leaving only a 'pocket-money' allowance. This increases the feeling of dependency and puts the client in a trap. Once admitted into care by a social services department there will rarely be opportunities to move and become independent, even in the situation where improvement took place and was sustained. In fact, provision of suitable accommodation for the handicapped is a statutory duty on local authorities, but a tremendous amount of pressure has often to be exerted to get a social services department to fulfil its legal obligations.

In the last decade Area Health Authorities have been encouraged to set up units for young disabled persons. Some have responded and new units have been designed and built in several areas. These units, where they exist, would be the choice of many patients because the financial penalties are not so stringent as in accommodation provided by the social services departments. However, in many units, because of the difficulty in recruiting staff to look after the chronically handicapped, the original role of caring for the young, chronically sick has been diluted. Many beds have been turned over to supply short stay accommodation for the provision of holidays or while physiotherapy treatment is provided. In some units it has got to the point where there are, in fact, no long term beds available. This is not intended to decry the use of beds to provide short stay admissions and short periods of specific treatment. Neither is it to minimise the fact that recruiting the necessary staff is difficult if the task is solely to be that of looking after the chronically handicapped. But the result is that there is too little accommodation for the handicapped which they can look on as their home.

To have a chance of a satisfactory placement the patient needs to live near an existing unit, to be under the age of 55 and to be reasonably socially adaptable. Even when admitted to the unit problems do not cease because, in theory, at the age of 65 the patient should be transferred from the young chronic sick unit to the geriatric services. Thus a major upheaval is scheduled for a time in life when the patient is least able to tolerate it. For the large number of patients who become handicapped between the ages of 55 and 65 the prospect of satisfactory placement is bleak. Many end up inappropriately living in geriatric wards.

The social services departments and Health Authorities may choose to discharge their responsibility by paying for places in homes run by charities. Financial constraints then depend on the sponsoring body. The quality of care depends upon the charity. Enormous changes in the financial support of charities have taken place as most now rely on the social services departments and Health Authorities for a large part of their running costs.

Between the two World Wars, when many of the present charities flourished, there was little inflation. The cost of caring for residents was low and expectation minimal. The level of community and medical care was lower than today and many patients died earlier from infections and intercurrent illnesses.

Today the picture has changed. Increased staffing levels and shorter working hours have caused the cost of care to explode, and the general cost of care has increased with inflation. Long term care for many can take place within the community, so fewer patients with conditions such as arthritis are admitted. The improved quality of medical care, and the use of intensive treatment units has led to the survival of many brain-damaged patients who previously would have died. Genteel 'Palm Court' arthritics stay at home instead of coming into care. Now care is needed for multiple sclerosis, head injury and stroke victims. Many of the units are not prepared or able to cope with the changes of attitudes that are needed.

All those who have been involved in trying to place such patients will be well aware of the difficulties.

Different approaches to residential care

It is worth pursuing further the attitudes and problems which exacerbate the situation. Miller and Gwynne (1972) put forward a distressing analysis of long term care in which they suggest that two models exist. One is the '*horticultural*' model, the second the '*warehousing*' model.

In the *horticultural model* it is suggested that the handicapped should be assessed for their residual abilities. These should be fostered to leave as much as possible for the individuals themselves to do. Support would only be provided when essential and on a limited basis.

In the *warehousing model* residents are there to be got up, fed, clothed, put to bed. They are required to conform to a system which was designed primarily, if subconsciously, for the convenience or the egos of the staff. They suggest that a hierarchy would soon be established which was defensive of its own rights and status. This would sap the residents' individuality so that they became 'institutionalised'. This process can be seen in many units, where the zombie-like attitude and indifference of the residents is only too apparent. In fact it allows those who do the caring to use this as the justification for continuing it! In the units following the warehousing model innumerable excuses are put forward to justify the *status quo*. For example:

(a) '*Patients with multiple sclerosis get very tired, therefore they have to get to bed early*'. This gives licence to start putting patients to bed early. The real reason is not to do with the 'tiredness' of the patients but more the convenience of the staff rosters since there are fewer staff on duty during the evening when patients, given the choice, would prefer to go to bed.

(b) *'They can't help being incontinent, you know'*. This is used as an excuse to respond to the problems of incontinence with pads, urinals, catheters and so forth. The fact that immobility or lack of communication may be the cause of incontinence is not taken into account. In one unit the female toilets were only available for three brief sessions during the day. The reason given was that it was difficult to staff them. The 50 yard queue outside the toilets at each session was an eloquent testimony to the effect of this attitude on the residents.

(c) *'They can't think for themselves, you know'*. This may eventually be true for those who suffer the rigours of institutional care for many years, but it does not automatically apply and should not apply at the early stages when residents seek admission.

Resident participation in management is still a rarity, and the institutions' reluctance to experiment or innovate prevents the handicapped from gaining independence. If organisations became more *'client orientated'* some of the unpleasant attitudes seen today might diminish and greater independence be returned to the patients. This cannot be a one-sided process. Greater independence must mean more responsibility for the patient if the system is to work. Some units have been too client-orientated and the staff have felt threatened. It was assumed that all complaints made by the residents were valid, so the staff were in no position to impose any discipline. This might work in a perfect world, but in the one we have compromise seems inevitable. Modification of attitudes, better information and more sensible use of volunteers and staff could all make a substantial contribution to the welfare of the handicapped within our existing resources.

Over the last few years much has been done to improve community care. If all the statutory facilities are available and are used, it can give comprehensive support. Developed properly, the majority of seriously handicapped people could be cared for in their own homes.

Those in *long stay units* are less fortunate since their freedom of choice has been removed. There are, however, some interesting developments giving hope for the future.

Rehabilitation units and assessment units do exist which make every effort to get patients back from long stay care into the community. A unit run by Lambeth Social Services Department consists of a block of 35 purpose-built flats, each housing a family in which one or more members are handicapped. There is a small centre staffed day and night which provides cover and support where needed 24 hours a day. The centre also provides short stay residential care and a day centre, both primarily for assessment of handicap and the development of individual programmes which help other clients to cope. This has been a success in that a substantial proportion of clients have been able to leave long stay care and go into their own flats.

Over the last few years there has been a perceptible, and long overdue, change in the role of those who care, particularly volunteers (see chapter 8). In some units volunteers have been successfully involved in caring. They are able to give time at awkward hours, giving residents greater freedom in getting up and going to bed. They can escort residents out and contribute greatly to their social lives. Used constructively volunteers can be a tremendous asset. When they confine their role to that of Victorian patrons, however, it is not surprising that the residents feel patronised. If volunteers want status or a self-righteous glow from their efforts, they would do better to stay away and raise funds.

Recommendations

In the introduction to this chapter it was stated that at present the best provisions have to be made within the framework of existing knowledge, since there is as yet no cure in sight for the disease of multiple sclerosis.

Residential care is inevitable for some, so provision must be made for creating homely conditions and a positive atmosphere. Such accommodation could be based on the horticultural model and be remote from a hospital environment. They should be small and be able to assess the abilities of each resident. There should be facilities to retrain lost skills, and every encouragement should be made to restore as much independence as possible. No hospital hierarchy, uniform or titles should be necessary, although the relevant skills of therapists, social workers, nurses and doctors should be available when needed, as for an ordinary family. There should be no forced segregation of sexes. Facilities for travel, socialising and entertaining guests are essential. So also is privacy. Whenever possible residents should deal with their own medication, and where this is not possible other residents should be recruited to help the less able. Such units should be managed by the residents and the staff equally. It has to be recognised that the staff will need support so that they do not feel vulnerable and threatened by the intransigent resident. (They do exist!)

Such homes could also give support to the handicapped in the local community, and help potential residents to look to their local home as a centre for advice, help and friendship. It would make a later move into residence there an easier step to make. Nothing about this is revolutionary. It already happens in some few homes in the United Kingdom and overseas. The major problem is to encourage the progressive attitudes already established to become standard practice.

It is, however, not just a problem for those who provide care. Eventually it will develop from an enlightened attitude to care from staff, residents, and from the general population. To be successful all need to be better informed and more tolerant. Conferences are one of the crucial catalysts in bringing about the general changes so desperately needed.

References

Miller, E. J. and Gwynne, G. V. (1972). *A Life Apart*, Tavistock Publications, London.

Postscript: The future

Rudy Capildeo and Audrey Maxwell

There is a lot of evidence to support our view that research into multiple sclerosis has reached an important and exciting stage (see chapter 1). Many research workers believe that the discovery of an aetiological agent is imminent. This must be tempered by the evidence that the disease does seem to be multifactorial: age, sex, heredity and geography all appear to be important. If the disease is due to a virus, is it a well known virus or is it a new type of virus? Whatever the research workers find in the next few years, the question will still be asked, 'What does it mean to the patient who already has the disease?'

In medicine, we alway think of the patient. Our approach may differ depending upon our discipline. For this reason, an interdisciplinary team, like the rehabilitation team, combines the skills of the different disciplines. Individual skills are important but the team approach, the overlapping of skills and the concerted effort for the patient's well-being are the most important aspects. As we learn more about multiple sclerosis we should inform our patients, their families and friends. It is important to involve them in their illness and to achieve a position of shared responsibility for it. Attitude of mind or motivation is vital for all concerned. Patients may openly or secretly hope for a 'cure'. From our understanding of the nature of multiple sclerosis this is unlikely, particularly if the agent is virus-like and persists in the patient's system. Yet if we look at the problem in a different way then there is much more hope.

One of the features of the disease is the pattern of remissions and relapses. Many patients may have difficulty in deciding what is a relapse. A very common complaint is the day to day variability, particularly the feeling of tiredness. If this picture is due to the individual's response to the causative agent (assuming that it is a persisting virus-like infection), then it might be possible to prevent further relapses by either stimulating the immune system or suppressing it - we do not yet know which would be more appropriate. This would give the central nervous system time to recover and, remembering how well many patients recover after an acute attack, this might mean no further attacks. Furthermore, it might be possible to immunise the population against multiple sclerosis, that is, to eradicate the disease. If this hypothesis is correct, then treatment for the new patient and the patient who has had the disease for many years will be equally important. The chance to prevent relapses will mean an improved quality of life. This is our hope for the future for our patients with multiple sclerosis.

Finally, in a time of recession we must consider the specialty of 'Rehabilitation'. In the United States of America, Europe and Scandinavia, 'rehabilitation' is considered to be a separate specialty for medical training; this is not the case in the United Kingdom. While this situation persists, the rehabilitation facilities for patients will continue to be woefully inadequate considering the country as a whole. Our hope for the future is that we can offer all our patients, wherever they live, access to a rehabilitation unit and the expertise of a rehabilitation team.

Author Index

Subject Index